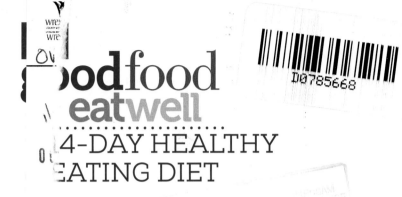

good food
eat well
14-DAY HEALTHY EATING DIET

10 9 8 7 6 5 4 3 2 1

BBC Books, an imprint of Ebury Publishing
20 Vauxhall Bridge Road,
London SW1V 2SA

BBC Books is part of the Penguin Random House group of companies, whose addresses can be found at
global.penguinrandomhouse.com

Penguin
Random House
UK

Photographs © BBC Worldwide, 2015
Recipes © BBC Worldwide, 2015
Book design © BBC Worldwide, 2015

First published by BBC Books in 2015

www.eburypublishing.co.uk

A CIP catalogue record for this book is available from the British Library

ISBN 9781849909013

Printed and bound by Firmengruppe APPL, aprinta druck, Wemding, Germany
Colour origination by Dot Gradations Ltd, UK

Commissioning editor: Lizzy Gray
Editorial manager: Lizzy Gaisford
Project editor: Helena Caldon
Designers: Interstate Creative Partners Ltd
Design manager: Kathryn Gammon
Production: Alex Goddard

Penguin Random House is committed to a sustainable future
for our business, our readers and our planet. This book is made
from Forest Stewardship Council® certified paper.

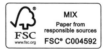

MIX
Paper from
responsible sources
FSC® C004592
www.fsc.org

PICTURE AND RECIPE CREDITS

BBC *Good Food* magazine and BBC Books would like to thank the following people for providing photos. While every effort has
been made to trace and acknowledge all photographers, we should like to apologize should there be any errors or omissions.

Peter Cassidy p97, p129, p135, p155, p159; Will Heap p19, p69, p85, p115, p123, p127; Lara Holmes p53, p87, p137; Adrian
Lawrence p73, p83; Gareth Morgans p167, p181; David Munns p95, p111, p173, p177; Myles New p57, p131, p147, p171, p187; Lis
Parsons p121, p183; Michael Paul p169; Craig Robertson p185; Howard Shooter p113; Maja Smend p179; Roger Stowell p175; Sam
Stowell p25, p27, p31, p33, p35, p51, p55, p61, p67, p71, p75, p77, p79, p93, p99, p101, p103, p105, p107, p109, p117, p119, p125,
p133, p139, p141, p145, p149, p151, p153, p157, p161, p163, p165; Rob Streeter p21, p29, p37, p39, p41, p43, p45, p47, p49, p59,
p63, p65, p89, p91, p143; Philip Webb p81.

All the recipes in this book were created by the editorial team at *Good Food* and by regular contributors to BBC magazines.

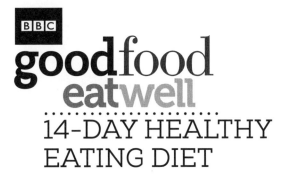

BBC goodfood eatwell
14-DAY HEALTHY EATING DIET

Editor **Sara Buenfeld**

BOOKS

Contents

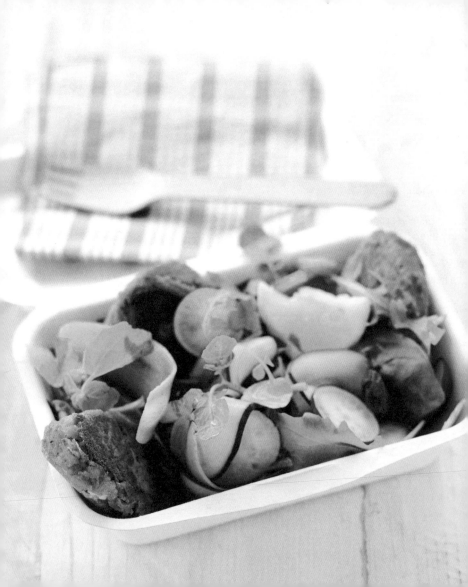

Introduction

If you want to make positive changes to your health and the way you feel, simple adjustments to your diet and lifestyle can reap benefits. Eat the right things and you will feel re-energised, and you may even see some welcome weight loss – especially if you move more too. Even little things help, such as walking up the stairs, instead of taking the escalator, or taking the dog for a walk.

However, many of us need a little nudge and some inspiration to set us on the right path, and that is where this handy little book comes in. Created from *BBC Good Food* magazine recipes, you will find a wealth of healthy dishes for breakfast, lunch and evening meals, plus a two-week healthy-eating plan that has been devised to flood your body with all the right nutrients to get you started.

Each recipe has been analysed on a per-serving basis, so you can see exactly what each dish contains – from the calories, fat and sugar right down to the salt quantities. And Kerry Torrens, *Good Food*'s nutritional therapist, has given you all the information that you need over the next few pages to make the right choices, with tips on portion size and snacking as well as advice to help you break bad habits.

The recipes in the book mostly cater for one or two portions; dishes that serve more are suitable for freezing or storing in the fridge for a few days, or are meals for entertaining. The desserts section should be used only occasionally, as a treat.

Sara

Sara Buenfeld
BBC Good Food magazine

How the diet plan works

Our two-week diet plan is a well-balanced one. None of the major food groups has been left out, so the plan will give your body a boost of nutritionally rich food, from fresh fruit and veg to lean protein, healthy fats, wholegrains and fibre, and ensure that you stay well hydrated.

The focus is on a low-GI way of eating, so you get enough of the right kind of carbs balanced with lean sources of protein in every meal and snack. This way of eating helps stabilise energy, keeps you fuller longer and avoids the need for those mid-afternoon sugar fixes that can cause erratic energy levels.

What's more, the diet is packed with foods rich in vital vitamins – including the B group – and the mineral chromium, which both work to stabilise blood-sugar levels to keep you energised. We've not forgotten the essential fats either, such as the omega-3 variety found in oily fish, nuts and seeds, which boost levels of the brain-chemical serotonin that governs your appetite and mood.

And did you know, your digestion isn't just about breaking down food to supply the energy you need? It also manages how acid or alkaline your body is. The ideal is an alkaline environment because then all the functions of the body work best. So we've ensured plenty of alkalising plant-based recipes to keep your body functioning at its peak and to keep you fighting fit. So if you are not already a vegetarian you can look forward to some delicious veggie dishes to complement the meat in your diet.

What you should be eating

Where possible, opt for quality produce – preferably ingredients that are in season and can be sourced from local suppliers – that way you can ensure what you eat is as fresh as possible and at its best nutritionally.

Lean proteins – whether you're a meat eater or not, good sources of lean protein are essential. Opt for lean cuts like pork fillet, skinless chicken and turkey as well as white and oily fish, beans, pulses, dairy and eggs.
Healthy oils – olive, rapeseed and flaxseed are all you'll need for healthy cooking, dressings and drizzles. Natural fats found in oily fish (salmon, trout, tuna, sardines and mackerel) as well as raw

nuts, seeds and olives are the most beneficial to your diet. Choose good-quality cold-pressed oils for dressings and drizzles, but don't cook with them because high temperatures can cause these delicate oils to lose their nutritional value. Use rapeseed instead, which is stable at high temperatures.

Fruit and veg – aim for a minimum of five different fruit and vegetables each day; pile your plate with a riot of different colours to ensure you get the mix of protective antioxidants you need. Fill up on veg while opting for lower-sugar fruits such as grapefruit, green apples and cranberries. To ring the changes, or to save time, you can also include frozen fruit and veg.

Good carbs – Ditch the white carbs and processed 'treats' – they may have great appeal but you'll get more energy from wholegrain pasta, brown rice, rye, spelt and quinoa. So, forget the energy bars that are typically full of refined sugars and instead stick to clean, unprocessed wholefoods that satisfy your energy need (see our snack suggestions p10).

Herbs and spices – an ideal way to help cut the salt, adding herbs and spices to your recipes may also aid digestion, help with blood-sugar balance and even fire up your metabolism.

5 WAYS TO GET THE MOST FROM OUR PLAN

Mindful munching – be aware of what, where and how you eat. Experts believe we eat 200–300 calories a day unconsciously.

Know your food – read labels. It's easy to become detached when we're not aware of what's in packaged foods like cereal, for example. Look out for hidden salt, sugar and saturated fats.

Be active – combine our vitality plan with 30 minutes' brisk exercise each day to maximise results. Try walking, cycling, dancing – anything that gets you warmer and a little out of breath. *If you're new to exercise, check with your GP before starting a regime.*

Hydrate – staying hydrated keeps you alert and helps control your appetite. Aim to drink 6–8 cups of fluid a day. Tea and coffee count, but it's best not to rely on them, so enjoy water, herbal teas and juices too. If you're at a desk all day, keep a glass of water to hand.

Get a good night – lack of sleep disrupts appetite hormones and can lead to carb cravings.

KNOW YOUR WEAKNESSES

It's easy to make occasional bad choices; these are the ones to watch out for:

Latte on the way to work – break the habit by opting for a green tea, or change your route so you avoid the coffee shop.

Mid-afternoon lifter – by 3 or 4 o'clock most of us are flagging and looking for that quick fix. Move the biscuit barrel out of sight and put fruit where you can see it, or reach for one of our suggested snacks (see below) for a healthier option. Never eat bought snacks directly out of the packet – just pour out a single serving and stick to it.

Relaxing tipple – most of us enjoy a glass of wine, but be aware of the Government guidelines and know exactly how much a unit is. Each week set aside at least 2 days, preferably consecutive, to be alcohol-free. If you do fancy a drink, make it a glass of red – Cabernet Sauvignon, Petite Syrah and Pinot Noir are said to have among the highest levels of the protective antioxidant resveratrol. For more information see www.drinkaware.co.uk/check-the-facts/what-is-alcohol.

Good-for-you snacks

All of the following are good healthy choices that will keep your blood sugars topped up until your next meal.

- Portion of cheese, such as Edam, with a pear or an apple
- Two plums with a cupped handful (25g/1oz) of unsalted nuts or seeds – almonds, walnuts or pumpkin seeds
- A small carton of low-fat Greek yogurt topped with frozen berries
- 1 apple sliced and dipped in peanut butter (with no added sugar)
- 1 tbsp houmous with strips of veggies
- 2–3 dried apricots with a couple of Brazil nuts
- 2 oatcakes topped with guacamole and salsa
- 2 squares (about 25g/1oz) of 70% cocoa solids dark chocolate
- 25g/1oz homemade popcorn sprinkled with ground cinnamon or chilli
- A slice of rye bread topped with cottage cheese and slices of pear
- Avocado & strawberry smoothie (page 46)
- Minty pineapple smoothies (page 48)

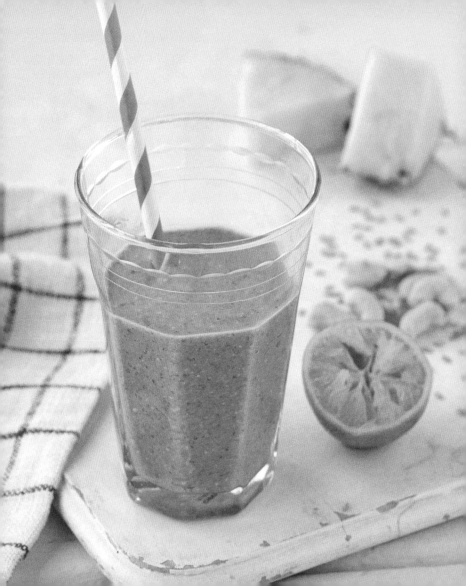

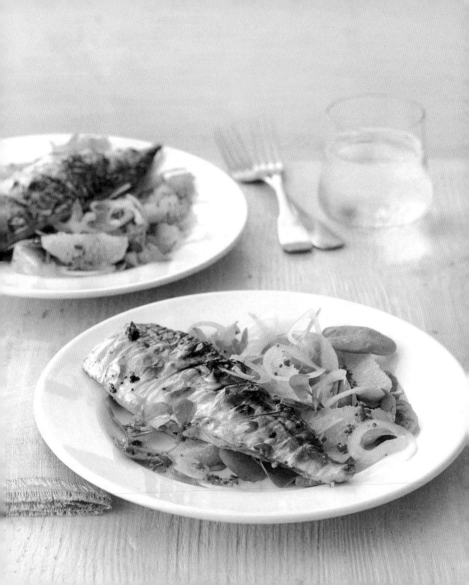

Your 14-day healthy eating plan

Per week, this plan includes at least five portions of fruit and vegetables a day, lots of meat-free options, at least 2 portions of fish (one being oily), as well as plenty of wholegrains, nuts and seeds. We have also kept an eye on salt and sugar levels. These are just the basic meals – we haven't included fruit, snacks or milk for tea as this isn't a weight-loss diet where you are counting calories.

Think about portion sizes

Choose a plate that holds the amount of food you can fit into your cupped hands. This represents the size of a main meal that best meets your needs. Next, divide the plate into quarters – fill one with protein, the second with healthy low-GI carbs and the other two with vegetables and salad.

Here's how a portion looks:

Protein (poultry, lean meat, eggs, fish, dairy and veggie alternatives like tofu) – the size of the palm of your hand; for cheese the equivalent of two of your fingers

Carbs (brown rice, pasta, bread and potatoes) – about the size of your clenched fist

Fat (butter/spreads) – the size of your thumbnail

All the recipes in this book are analysed on their listed ingredients only, excluding optional extras such as serving suggestions or seasoning – and so these quantities are not included. If you serve the portion sizes suggested, you can work out how each recipe fits into your day-to-day diet by comparing the figures with the Reference Intake (RI). These are the recommended daily figures based on an average adult for the amount of energy (kilocalories), fat, saturated fat, carbohydrate, sugar, protein and salt an average adult should consume each day.

Reference Intake (RI). The figures below for fat, saturated fat, sugar and salt are maximum daily amounts and so should not be exceeded.

Energy (Kilocalories): 2,000
Protein: 50g
Carbohydrate: 260g
Sugar: 90g
Fat: 70g
Saturated fat: 20g
Salt: 6g

Week 1

MON	Breakfast	Creamy porridge with apple & raisin compote (p32)
	Lunch	Mushroom & basil omelette (p62)
	Evening meal	Squash, mushroom & gorgonzola pilaf (p144)
TUES	Breakfast	Fig & seed bread (p40)
	Lunch	Spicy turkey tabbouleh (p50)
	Evening meal	Baked potatoes with spicy dhal (p138) with salad
WED	Breakfast	Porridge with pear, cinnamon & walnuts (p30)
	Lunch	Asparagus soup (p80)
	Evening meal	Lamb with buckwheat noodles (p156)
THURS	Breakfast	Berry pancake (p22)
	Lunch	Turkey, pea guacamole & radish wrap (p52)
	Evening meal	Salsa spaghetti with sardines (p118)
FRI	Breakfast	Avocado & strawberry smoothie (p46)
	Lunch	Asparagus salad with a runny poached egg (p64)
	Evening meal	Piri-piri fish & chips with spicy peas (p124)
SAT	Breakfast	Creamy porridge with apple & raisin compote (p32)
	Lunch	Mini spinach & cottage-cheese frittatas (p86) with salad
	Evening meal	Seared steak with celery & pepper caponata (p160)
SUN	Breakfast	Baked-eggs brunch (p18)
	Lunch	Tuna, avocado & pea salad in Baby Gem lettuce (p58)
	Evening meal	Herb roast pork with vegetable roasties (p164)

Week 2

MON	Breakfast	Vanilla-almond chia breakfast bowl (p36)
	Lunch	Fattoush (p84)
	Evening meal	Cajun grilled chicken (p88)
TUES	Breakfast	Fig & seed bread (p40)
	Lunch	Chickpea patties with carrot & raisin salad (p78)
	Evening meal	Citrus & ginger steamed fish with stir-fry veg (p132)
WED	Breakfast	Pistachio nut & spiced apple bircher (p38)
	Lunch	Curried egg-mayo open sandwich (p70)
	Evening meal	Aubergine tagine (p148)
THURS	Breakfast	Rye bread with almond butter & pink grapefruit (p44)
	Lunch	Courgette tortilla with toppings (p66)
	Evening meal	Tasty turkey meatballs (p104)
FRI	Breakfast	Berry pancake (p22)
	Lunch	Pepper & walnut houmous (p76)
	Evening meal	Fresh salmon trout with new potato & watercress salad (p116)
SAT	Breakfast	Smoky rashers & tomatoes on toast (p24)
	Lunch	Egg & veggie pittas (p68)
	Evening meal	Fragrant spiced chicken with banana sambal (p98)
SUN	Breakfast	Poached eggs with smoked salmon & bubble & squeak (p20)
	Lunch	Moroccan-roasted veg soup (p82)
	Evening meal	Lemon & garlic roast chicken (p90)

Notes &
conversion tables

· ·

NOTES ON THE RECIPES
- Eggs are large in the UK and Australia and extra large in America unless stated.
- Wash fresh produce before preparation.
- Recipes contain nutritional analyses for 'sugar', which means the total sugar content including all natural sugars in the ingredients, unless otherwise stated.

OVEN TEMPERATURES

GAS	°C	°C FAN	°F	OVEN TEMP.
¼	110	90	225	Very cool
½	120	100	250	Very cool
1	140	120	275	Cool or slow
2	150	130	300	Cool or slow
3	160	140	325	Warm
4	180	160	350	Moderate
5	190	170	375	Moderately hot
6	200	180	400	Fairly hot
7	220	200	425	Hot
8	230	210	450	Very hot
9	240	220	475	Very hot

APPROXIMATE WEIGHT CONVERSIONS
- All the recipes in this book list both metric and imperial measurements. Conversions are approximate and have been rounded up or down. Follow one set of measurements only; do not mix the two.
- Cup measurements, which are used in Australia and America, have not been listed here as they vary from ingredient to ingredient. Kitchen scales should be used to measure dry/solid ingredients.

Good Food is concerned about sustainable sourcing and animal welfare. Where possible, humanely reared meats, sustainably caught fish (see fishonline.org for further information from the Marine Conservation Society) and free-range chickens and eggs are used when recipes are originally tested.

SPOON MEASURES

Spoon measurements are level unless otherwise specified.
- 1 teaspoon (tsp) = 5ml
- 1 tablespoon (tbsp) = 15ml
- 1 Australian tablespoon = 20ml (cooks in Australia should measure 3 teaspoons where 1 tablespoon is specified in a recipe)

APPROXIMATE LIQUID CONVERSIONS

METRIC	IMPERIAL	AUS	US
50ml	2fl oz	¼ cup	¼ cup
125ml	4fl oz	½ cup	½ cup
175ml	6fl oz	¾ cup	¾ cup
225ml	8fl oz	1 cup	1 cup
300ml	10fl oz/½ pint	½ pint	1¼ cups
450ml	16fl oz	2 cups	2 cups/1 pint
500ml	20fl oz/1 pint	1 pint	2½ cups
1 litre	35fl oz/1¾ pints	1¾ pints	1 quart

Baked-eggs brunch

· ·

Set yourself up for the day with a good breakfast of spinach, eggs, leeks and sun-dried tomatoes. Low in calories and meat-free, it's the perfect start to a busy weekend.

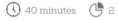 40 minutes 2

- 1 tbsp rapeseed oil
- 1 leek, thinly sliced
- 1 onion, thinly sliced
- 100g bag baby leaf spinach
- small handful fresh wholemeal breadcrumbs
- 15g/½oz Parmesan (or vegetarian alternative), finely grated
- 2 sun-dried tomatoes, chopped
- 2 medium eggs

1 Heat oven to 200C/180C fan/gas 6. Heat the oil in a pan and add the leek, onion and some seasoning. Cook for 15 minutes until soft and beginning to caramelise.

2 Meanwhile, put the spinach in a colander and pour over a kettle of boiling water. When cool enough to handle, squeeze out as much liquid as possible. Mix the breadcrumbs and cheese together.

3 Spoon the leek-and-onion mixture into two ovenproof dishes, then scatter with the spinach and pieces of sun-dried tomato. Make a well in the middle of each dish and crack an egg in it. Season and sprinkle with the cheese crumbs. Put the dishes on a baking sheet and cook in the oven for 12–15 minutes, until the whites of the eggs are set and the yolks are cooked to your liking and ready to serve.

· ·

PER SERVING 225 kcals, protein 12g, carbs 10g, fat 13g, sat fat 3g, fibre 5g, sugar 7g, salt 0.5g

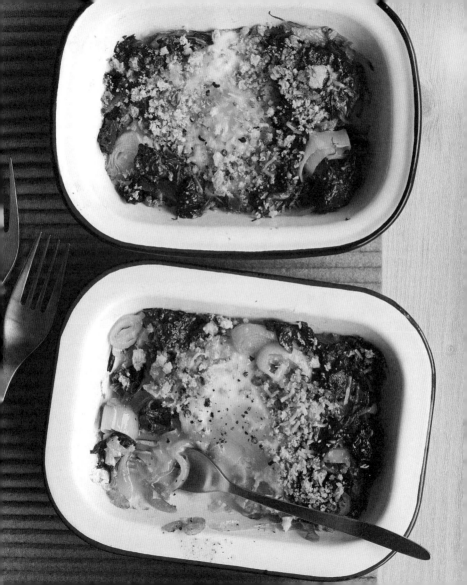

Poached eggs with smoked salmon & bubble & squeak

· ·

Although salmon is an oily fish, and so contains omega-3, the smoked version can be very salty and should be used sparingly.

🕐 20 minutes   🍽 2

- 300g/10oz whole new potatoes
- 1 tbsp rapeseed oil
- 140g/5oz white cabbage, finely chopped
- 2 spring onions, finely sliced
- 1 tbsp snipped chives
- 2 medium eggs, at room temperature
- 75g/2½oz smoked salmon

1 Cook the potatoes in a pan of boiling water for about 15 minutes until tender, then drain.

2 Heat the oil in a non-stick frying pan or wok. Add the cabbage and the spring onions, and cook for a couple of minutes. Meanwhile, chop and squash the potatoes roughly, then add to the pan or wok along with the chives. Cook for 4–5 minutes, flip it over (don't worry if it breaks) and cook for a further 4–5 minutes.

3 Meanwhile, bring a small pan of water to a rolling boil then reduce the heat so it is just simmering. Crack the eggs into the pan and cook for about 3 minutes until the whites are firm and the yolk is just beginning to set. Remove with a slotted spoon and drain on kitchen paper.

4 To serve, divide the bubble and squeak between two plates, put the smoked salmon and poached eggs on top and grind over a little black pepper, to taste.

· ·

PER SERVING 310 kcals, protein 19g, carbs 29g, fat 13g, sat fat 2g, fibre 4g, sugar 5g, salt 2g

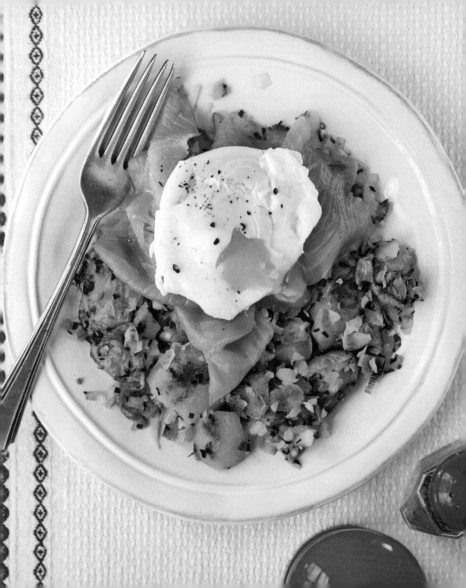

Berry pancake

This delicious high-protein breakfast is a one-egg omelette cleverly disguised as a pancake. Berries are naturally sweet, so you shouldn't need extra sweeteners.

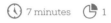 7 minutes 1

- 1 egg
- 1 tbsp skimmed milk
- 3 pinches ground cinnamon
- ½ tsp rapeseed oil
- 100g/4oz low-fat cottage cheese
- 175g/6oz mixed chopped strawberries, blueberries and raspberries

1 Beat the egg and milk with the cinnamon in a small bowl. Heat the rapeseed oil in a 20cm non-stick frying pan and pour in the egg mixture, swirling evenly to cover the base. Cook for a few minutes until set and golden underneath. There's no need to flip it over.

2 Put the eggy pancake on a plate, spread over the cottage cheese then scatter with the mixed chopped strawberries, blueberries and raspberries. Roll up and serve.

PER PANCAKE 264 kcals, protein 21g, carbs 18g, fat 12g, sat fat 4g, fibre 4g, sugar 16g, salt 1g

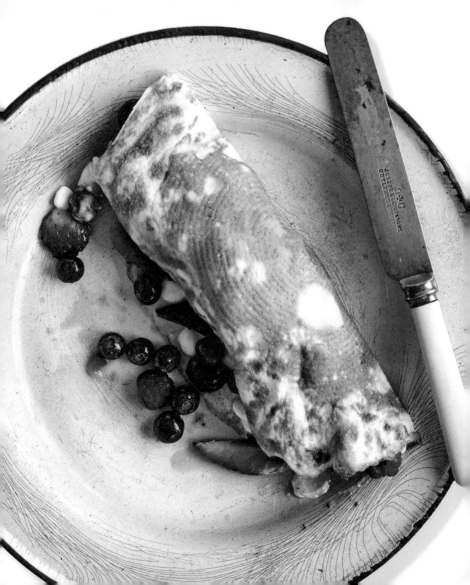

Smoky rashers & tomatoes on toast

Turkey rashers are a great low-fat alternative to bacon, while mashed avocado replaces the butter, contributing to a breakfast with two of your 5-a-day.

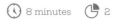 8 minutes   2

- rapeseed oil, for greasing
- 4 smoked turkey rashers
- 3 tomatoes, halved
- 2 slices wholewheat bread
- 1 tsp English mustard
- 1 small ripe avocado
- 2 handfuls rocket leaves

1 Heat a non-stick pan or griddle and spray or rub with a little oil lightly to grease it. Cook the turkey rashers and tomatoes for a couple of minutes each side.

2 Meanwhile, toast the bread, spread with mustard and squash half an avocado on top. Pile on the turkey rashers and tomatoes with the rocket and serve while still hot.

PER SERVING 269 kcals, protein 19g, carbs 19g, fat 13g, sat fat 3g, fibre 6g, sugar 6g, salt 1.7g

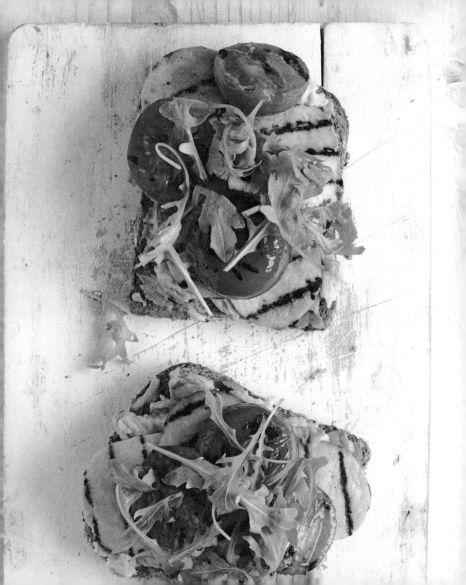

Creamy mustard mushrooms on toast served with orange juice

· ·

Serving this with a 150ml glass of fruit juice gains you a second portion of your 5-a-day. Even unsweetened juice like this is rich in natural sugars, so don't exceed it.

 10 minutes   1

- 1 slice wholemeal bread
- 1½ tbsp light soft cheese
- 1 tsp rapeseed oil
- 3 handfuls sliced small flat mushrooms
- 2 tbsp skimmed milk
- ¼ tsp wholegrain mustard
- 1 tbsp snipped chives
- 150ml/¼ pint orange juice, freshly squeezed or unsweetened from a carton

1 Toast the bread then spread with a little of the soft cheese instead of using butter.
2 Meanwhile, heat the oil in a non-stick pan, add the mushrooms and cook, stirring frequently, until they have softened.
3 Spoon in the milk, remaining cheese and the mustard, and stir well until coated. Tip on to the toast and top with the chives. Serve with a glass of orange juice.

· ·
PER SERVING 231 kcals, protein 13g, carbs 28g, fat 7g, sat fat 2g, fibre 4g, sugar 16g, salt 0.1g

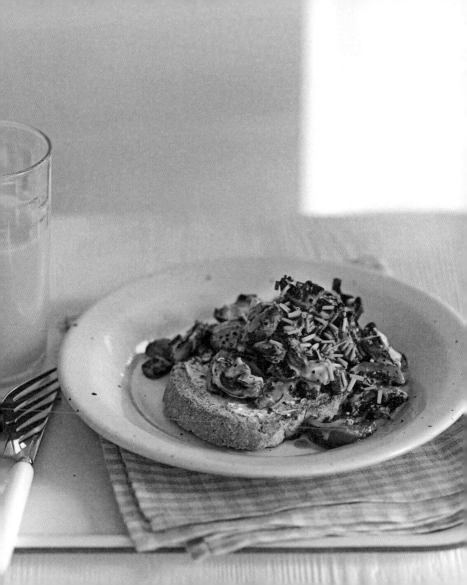

Eggy spelt bread with orange cheese & raspberries

Try this French toast with a healthy twist. Use spelt or wholemeal bread and top with light, citrusy cottage cheese and your favourite fresh seasonal fruit.

🕐 10 minutes   🍽 2

- 2 medium eggs
- 2 tbsp unsweetened orange juice
- 2 slices spelt bread, halved
- 1 tsp rapeseed oil
- 50g/2oz low-fat cottage cheese
- 1 tsp orange zest
- 50g/2oz raspberries
- clear honey, to drizzle (optional)

1 Beat the eggs and orange juice in a bowl wide enough to fit the bread in it. Soak the bread in the eggs and juice for 2 minutes or so, turning halfway through.

2 Put the rapeseed oil in a non-stick frying pan over a high heat. When hot, add the eggy bread. Leave to cook for a couple of minutes undisturbed, then flip and cook on the other side for another 1–2 minutes.

3 Divide the bread between two plates, dollop the cottage cheese on top and sprinkle with the orange zest. Top with the raspberries and a drizzle of honey, if you like.

PER SERVING 124 kcals, protein 4g, carbs 23g, fat 3g, sat fat none, fibre 3g, sugar 1g, salt 0.16g

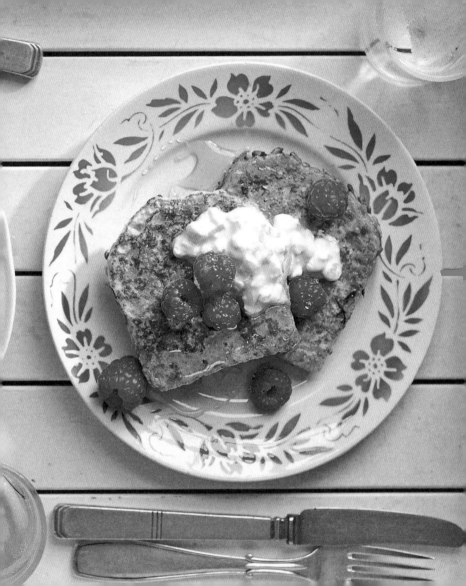

Porridge with pear, cinnamon & walnuts

· ·

If your cholesterol level is high, regularly eating oats can help reduce it. To vary the flavours stir in a small mashed banana with the yogurt, or top with raspberries.

🕐 10 minutes 🍽 1

- 3 tbsp porridge oats
- 150g pot 0%-fat probiotic natural yogurt
- 1 ripe pear, cored, skin left on and sliced
- few pinches ground cinnamon
- small handful roughly chopped walnuts

1 Tip 200ml/7fl oz water into a small non-stick pan, stir in the oats and cook over a low heat until bubbling and thickened. You can make this in a microwave, but use a deep container to prevent spillage because the mixture will rise up as it cooks. It will take 3 minutes on High.

2 Stir in the yogurt, spoon into a bowl then top with the pear, cinnamon and walnuts.

· ·
PER SERVING 341 kcals, protein 16g, carbs 41g, fat 12g, sat fat 1g, fibre 8g, sugar 27g, salt 0.4g

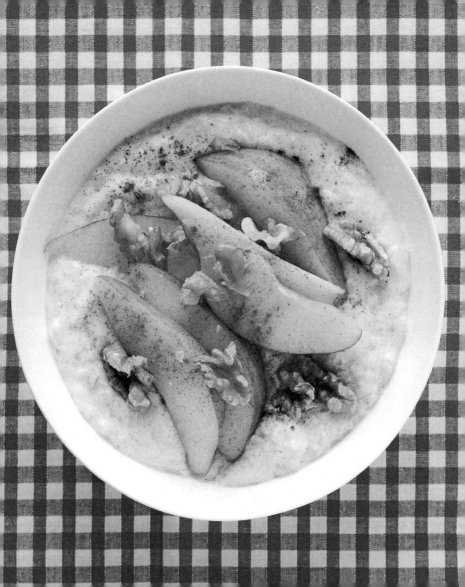

Creamy porridge with apple & raisin compote

· ·

This compote kick-starts your day with two of your 5-a-day. If mornings are a rush, make it the night before and serve chilled, or make it fresh and enjoy it warm.

🕐 15 minutes   👐 2

- 50g/2oz porridge oats
- 2 x 150g pots 0%-fat probiotic natural yogurt
- ½ handful sunflower seeds (optional)

FOR THE COMPOTE
- 2 dessert apples, peeled and thickly sliced
- 25g/1oz raisins
- 150ml/¼ pint orange juice

1 To make the compote, poach the apples in a covered pan with the raisins and orange juice for 8–10 minutes until the apples are tender. Mash a little of the apple to thicken the juice.

2 Meanwhile, make the porridge. Pour 400ml/14fl oz water into a non-stick pan, stir in the oats and cook over a low heat until bubbling and thickened. Take off the heat and stir in the yogurt.

3 Spoon the porridge into bowls then serve with the warm or cold compote and scatter with sunflower seeds, if you like.

· ·

PER SERVING 323 kcals, protein 16g, carbs 50g, fat 6g, sat fat 1g, fibre 5g, sugar 35g, salt 0.4g

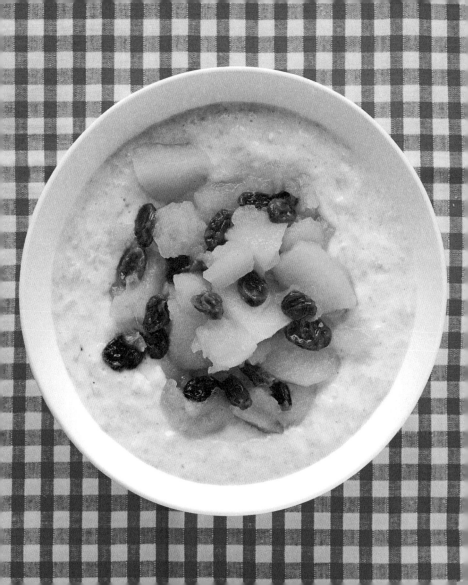

Apricot ginger & grapefruit compote

This is really zingy and refreshing, perfect with probiotic yogurt or porridge. The recipe makes enough to serve three, but it keeps in the fridge for a few days.

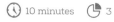 10 minutes 3

- 300g can breakfast apricots
- 1 tsp finely grated fresh ginger
- 2 pink grapefruits, peeled and cut into segments
- ½ handful sunflower seeds or flaked almonds, to serve (optional)

1 Tip the apricots and their juice into a bowl, add the ginger then blitz half the mixture with a stick blender to purée it and turn the juice into more of a sauce. Stir in the grapefruit segments and chill until ready to serve.
2 Use to top porridge or serve with yogurt and scatter over some sunflower seeds or almonds for some crunch, if you like.

PER SERVING 171 kcals, protein 4g, carbs 42g, fat 3g, sat fat 1g, fibre 2g, sugar 17g, salt 0.4g

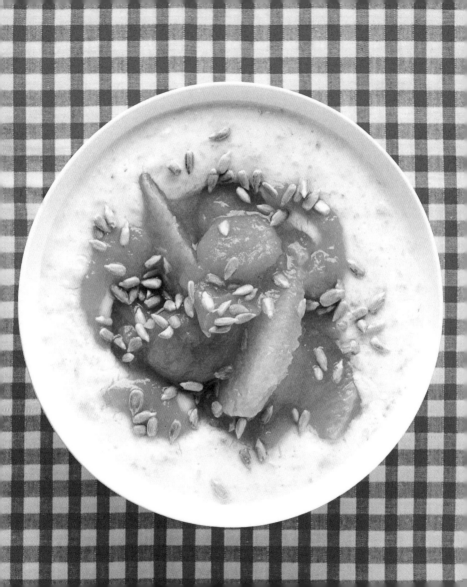

Vanilla-almond chia breakfast bowl

This fibre-packed oat pot is similar to a bircher. The combination of oats, blueberries, yogurt, omega-3-rich chia seeds and nuts will keep you full until lunchtime.

🕐 5 minutes, plus soaking   🥧 2

FOR THE PORRIDGE
- 50g/2oz jumbo porridge oats
- 200ml/7fl oz unsweetened almond milk
- ½ tsp vanilla extract
- 2 tbsp 0%-fat probiotic natural yogurt
- 25g/1oz chia seeds

FOR THE TOPPING
- 150g punnet blueberries
- 25g/1oz almonds, slivered or flaked
- clear honey, to taste (optional)

1 Mix all the porridge ingredients in a bowl and leave to soak for at least 20 minutes. Once the oats have softened, stir through half the blueberries. If the mixture is too dry, add a little water.

2 Divide the porridge between two bowls and top each with the remaining berries, the almonds and a drizzle of honey, if using, to taste.

PER SERVING 322 kcals, protein 11g, carbs 32g, fat 14g, sat fat 2g, fibre 10g, sugar 13g, salt 0.3g

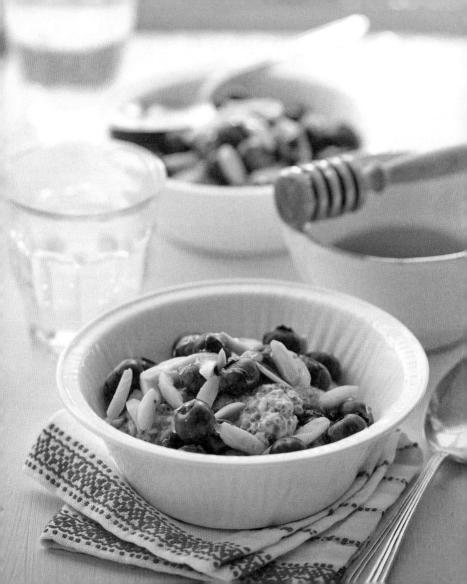

Pistachio nut & spiced-apple bircher

· ·

A balanced, filling breakfast bowl of oats and apple in low-fat yogurt spiced with cinnamon and nutmeg, topped with crunchy pomegranate seeds or juicy berries.

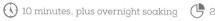 10 minutes, plus overnight soaking   2

FOR THE MUESLI BASE
- 50g/2oz jumbo porridge oats
- 50ml/2fl oz unsweetened apple juice
- large pinch ground cinnamon
- large pinch ground nutmeg
- 1 medium apple, cored and grated
- 2 tbsp 0%-fat probiotic natural yogurt

FOR THE TOPPING
- 25g/1oz chopped pistachio nuts
- 3 tbsp pomegranate seeds or mixed berries

1 Mix all the muesli base ingredients, except the yogurt, with 150ml/¼ pint water and leave to soak for at least 20 minutes or overnight, if possible.

2 Once the oats have softened, stir through the yogurt, then divide the mixture between two bowls.

3 Sprinkle half of the topping over each bowl and serve.

· ·
PER SERVING 229 kcals, protein 8g, carbs 29g, fat 8g, sat fat 1g, fibre 5g, sugar 14g, salt 0.1g

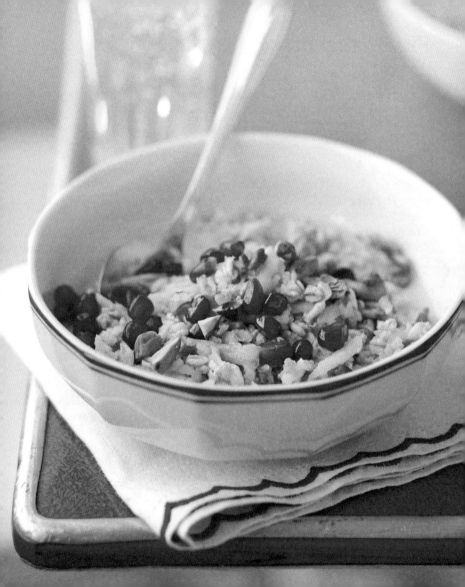

Fig & seed bread

Keep in the fridge, or cut slices for the freezer, for a great quick breakfast. Top with low-fat ricotta instead of butter and fresh fruit for a low-fat, high-protein alternative.

🕐 1½ hours   🍰 Cuts into 16

- 400ml/14fl oz hot strong black tea
- 100g/4oz dried figs, hard stalks removed, thinly sliced
- 140g/5oz sultanas
- 50g/2oz porridge oats
- 200g/7oz wholewheat self-raising flour
- 1 tsp baking powder
- 100g/4oz mixed nuts (almonds, walnuts, brazils, hazelnuts), plus 50g/2oz for the top
- 1 tbsp each golden linseed and sesame seeds, plus 2 tsp sesame seeds to sprinkle
- 25g/1oz pumpkin seeds
- 1 egg
- 25g/1oz ricotta
- thickly sliced orange or green apple, to top

1 Heat oven to 170C/150 fan/gas 3½. Pour the tea into a large bowl and stir in the figs, sultanas and oats. Set aside to soak while you get on with the rest of the loaf.

2 Line the base and sides of a 1kg loaf tin with baking parchment. Mix together the flour, baking powder, mixed nuts and the seeds. Beat the egg into the cooled fruit mixture then stir the dried ingredients into the wet.

3 Pile the mix into the tin then level the top and scatter with the remaining nuts and the sesame seeds.

4 Bake for 1 hour then cover the top with foil and bake for 15 minutes more until a skewer inserted into the centre of the loaf comes out clean. Remove from the tin to cool, but leave the baking parchment on until cold.

5 Serve sliced and spread with ricotta and topped with a slice of orange or apple. The bread will keep in the fridge for a month.

PER SERVING 249 kcals, protein 10g, carbs 30g, fat 10g, sat fat 3g, fibre 6g, sugar 20g, salt 0.3g

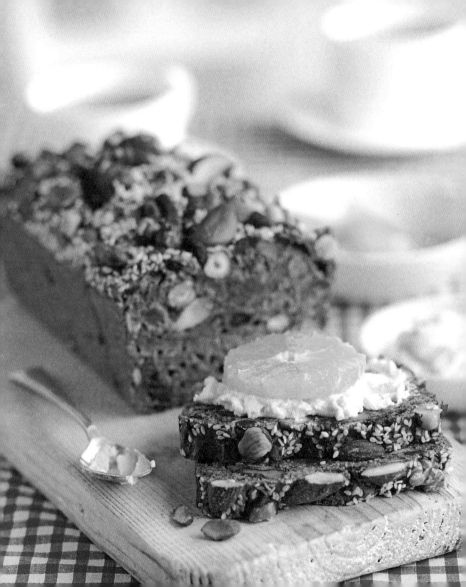

Almond nut butter

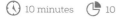

Blitz up your own homemade nut butter for spreading on toast for a speedy breakfast, filling pancakes or adding to sauces.

🕐 10 minutes   🥧 10

- 250g/9oz blanched almonds
- 2 tbsp mild oil, such as coconut, almond or olive oil

1 Put the almonds in a food processor and blitz on a high speed until finely chopped and the nuts have come together to form a thick ball. With the processor still running, add the oil, a little at a time, until the mixture is a smooth, glossy paste – about 7 minutes.

2 Spoon into a clean jar and keep tightly closed and chilled when not in use. Will keep in the fridge for up to 3 weeks.

PER SERVING 177 kcals, protein 5g, carbs 2g, fat 16g, sat fat 3g, fibre 2g, sugar 1g, salt none

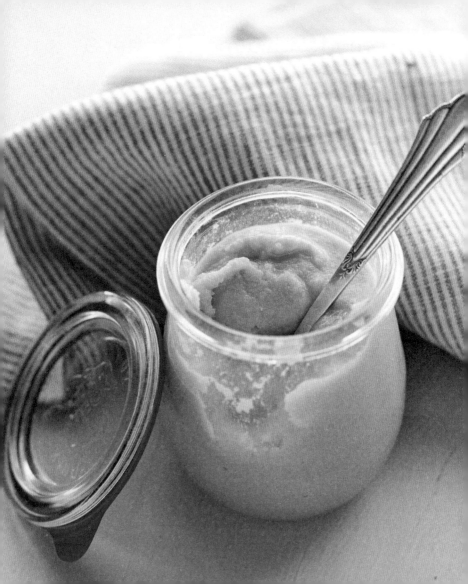

Rye bread with almond butter & pink grapefruit

A balanced breakfast of rye toast with homemade nut butter and juicy fruit.

🕐 5 minutes   🥧 2

- 2 slices rye bread
- 1 pink grapefruit
- 4 tbsp almond butter, bought or homemade (see page 42)

1 Toast the rye bread, if you like. Segment the grapefruit and spoon the fruit, along with any juice, into a small bowl.

2 Spread the almond butter on to the rye bread and top with the grapefruit segments, drizzling any juice over the top to serve.

PER SERVING 340 kcals, protein 10g, carbs 30g, fat 19g, sat fat 3g, fibre 8g, sugar 7g, salt 0.8g

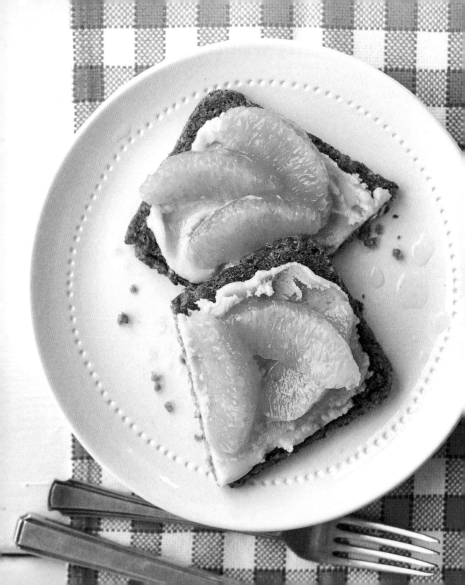

Avocado & strawberry smoothies

A creamy breakfast-friendly blend that's high in calcium and low in calories. You can serve this as a snack during the day too.

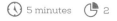 5 minutes   2

- ½ avocado, stoned, peeled and cut into chunks
- 150g/5½oz strawberries, halved
- 4 tbsp 0%-fat probiotic natural yogurt
- 200ml/7fl oz semi-skimmed milk
- lemon or lime juice and clear honey (optional), to taste

1 Put all the ingredients in a blender and whizz until smooth. If the consistency is too thick, add a little water. Divide between two glasses to serve.

PER SMOOTHIE 197 kcals, protein 9g, carbs 15g, fat 11g, sat fat 3g, fibre 3g, sugar 15g, salt 0.3g

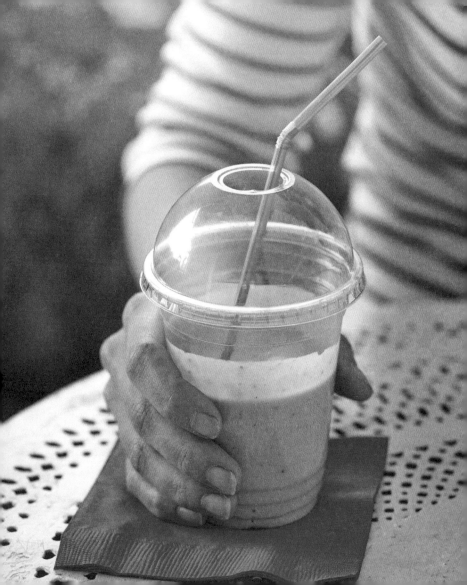

Minty pineapple smoothies

There's more to smoothies than fruit – this green blend contains spinach, oats, linseed and cashew nuts too. Serve for breakfast or eat as a snack.

🕐 10 minutes   🥧 2

- 200g/7oz pineapple, peeled, cored and cut into chunks
- a few mint leaves
- 50g/2oz baby leaf spinach
- 25g/1oz rolled oats
- 2 tbsp linseed
- handful unsalted unroasted cashew nuts
- lime juice, to taste

1 Put all the ingredients in a blender with 200ml/7fl oz water and process until smooth. If it's too thick, add more water (up to 400ml/14fl oz) until you get the right mix.
2 Adjust the lime juice to taste and pour into two glasses to serve.

PER SMOOTHIE 177 kcals, protein 6g, carbs 19g, fat 8g, sat fat 1g, fibre 4g, sugar 11g, salt 0.1g

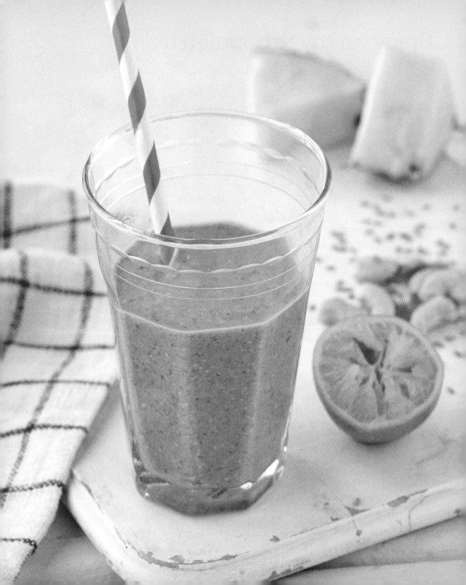

Spicy turkey tabbouleh

Turkey breast packs plenty of lean protein that will keep you fuller for longer. This tabbouleh salad of turkey and fresh salad ingredients is both delicious and satisfying.

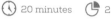 20 minutes 2

- 2 tbsp 0%-fat Greek yogurt
- 1 garlic clove, crushed
- ½ tsp smoked paprika
- juice ½ lemon
- 175g/6oz turkey breast chunks
- 50g/2oz bulghar wheat
- 1 small red onion, finely chopped
- 2 tomatoes, chopped
- ⅛ cucumber, diced
- 2 tbsp each chopped parsley and mint leaves

1 Heat the grill to high and line a baking sheet with foil. Mix together the yogurt, garlic, paprika and a squeeze of the lemon in a bowl then stir in the turkey. Arrange on the baking sheet.

2 Meanwhile, cook the bulghar according to the pack instructions then add all the remaining ingredients, including the rest of the lemon to make the tabbouleh.

3 Grill the turkey for 5–8 minutes and serve hot or cold with the tabbouleh salad. Keeps in the fridge for 2 days.

PER SERVING 224 kcals, protein 27g, carbs 24g, fat 2g, sat fat 0.3g, fibre 2g, sugar 5g, salt 0.2g

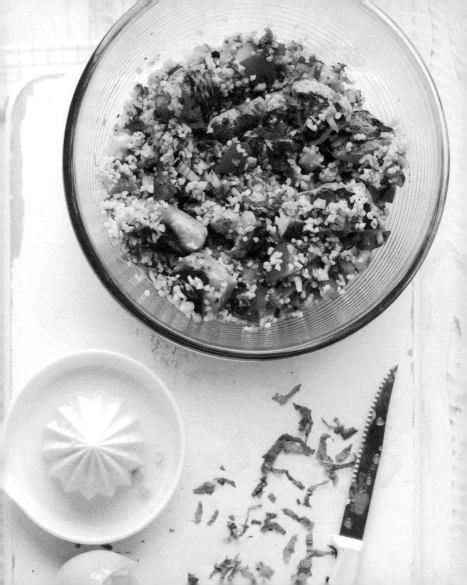

Turkey, pea-guacamole & radish wrap

Keep in shape with this lunchbox- and picnic-friendly wrap filled with lemony pea 'guacamole', low-fat soft cheese and lean white meat.

🕐 5 minutes 🥧 1

- 50g/2oz cold cooked peas
- 2 tbsp low-fat soft cheese
- a little lemon zest and juice
- 1 reduced-salt wrap
- 50g/2oz turkey, sliced
- 2–3 radishes, sliced

1 Crush the peas with the soft cheese and the lemon zest and juice, then season. Spread the guacamole over the wrap and top with the turkey slices and the radishes. Roll and cut in half and serve, wrapped in baking paper and tied with string to secure, if you like.

PER SERVING 339 kcals, protein 30g, carbs 32g, fat 9g, sat fat 4g, fibre 7g, sugar 6g, salt 1.2g

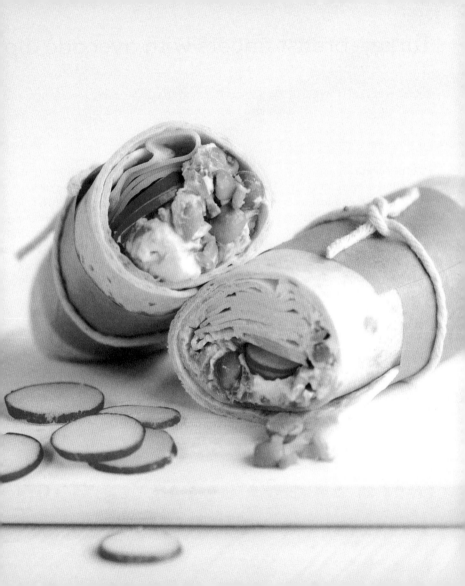

Turkey-breast fingers with avocado dip

Eat at home or take as a packed lunch for a midday boost. Avocados are packed with heart-healthy fats, protective vitamin E and glutathione, which protects brain cells.

🕐 15 minutes   🥧 2

FOR THE TURKEY
- 1 Oatibix or Weetabix
- 15g/½oz finely grated Parmesan
- ½ tsp each dried thyme and oregano
- 1 tsp each smoked paprika and ground coriander
- 344g pack turkey breast meat, cut into thick strips
- 1 egg, beaten
- cherry tomatoes, pomegranate seeds and salad leaves, to serve

FOR THE DIP
- 210g can butter beans, drained and rinsed
- 1 small avocado, stoned and peeled
- 4 spring onions, trimmed and chopped
- zest and juice 1 lime

1 Heat oven to 220C/200C fan/gas 7. Crumble the cereal into a shallow bowl then stir in the Parmesan, herbs and spices with a little seasoning. Dip the turkey into the beaten egg then coat with the cheesy spice mixture and lay on a baking sheet, spaced apart. Bake for 12 minutes.

2 Meanwhile, put the beans, avocado, spring onions, lime zest and juice in a bowl with some seasoning to make the dip and blitz with a hand blender until smooth.

3 Serve the dip with the hot or cold turkey and some cherry tomatoes, pomegranate seeds and salad leaves on the side.

PER SERVING 446 kcals, protein 54g, carbs 18g, fat 17g, sat fat 5g, fibre 6g, sugar 2g, salt 0.5g

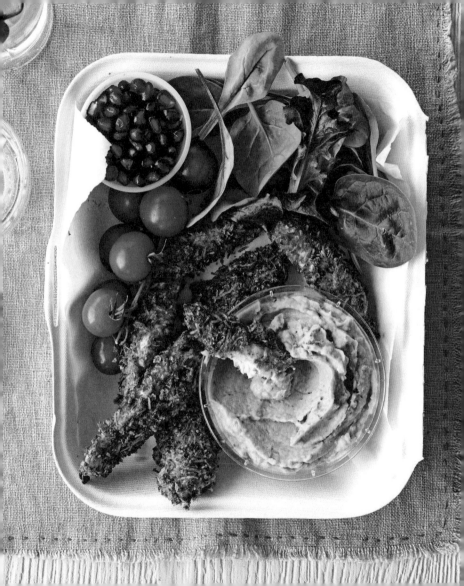

Chicken, lentil & sweetcorn chowder

· ·

A winter warmer without the calories. Try making double and freezing some for extra-quick lunches. If you want to serve some bread alongside, slice up some rye bread.

🕐 35 minutes 🥧 4

- 4 spring onions, trimmed and thinly sliced
- 850ml/1½ pints chicken stock
- 250g/9oz potatoes, diced
- 300ml/½ pint skimmed milk
- 250g/9oz boneless skinless chicken breast, cut into small pieces
- 140g/5oz frozen or canned sweetcorn
- 410g can Puy or green lentils, drained and rinsed
- snipped chives, to garnish (optional)

1 Put the spring onions in a large pan with 6 tablespoons of the stock and some seasoning. Cover and cook for 2–3 minutes until softened. Add the potatoes, the rest of the stock and the milk. Bring to the boil and simmer gently, partially covered, for 10 minutes or until the potatoes are just tender.

2 Ladle out about a quarter of the mixture into a blender and whizz until smooth. Stir back into the pan.

3 Add the chicken, sweetcorn and lentils to the pan, and cook for 5–7 minutes more or until the chicken is cooked. Check the seasoning and serve in warm bowls, scattered with snipped chives, if using.

· ·
PER SERVING 252 kcals, protein 31g, carbs 29g, fat 2g, sat fat 1g, fibre 6g, sugar 5g, salt 0.75g

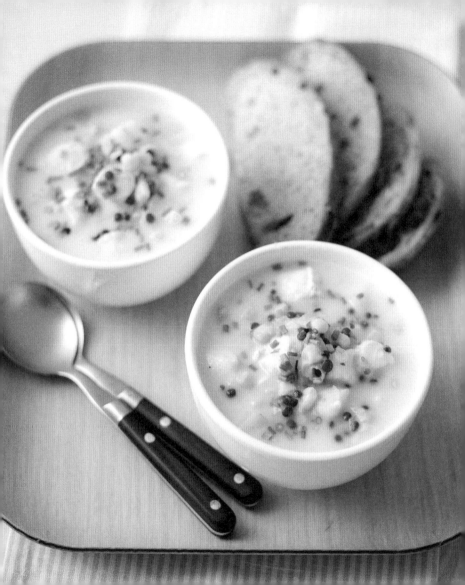

Tuna, avocado & pea salad in Baby Gem lettuce wraps

Skip the tortillas and serve a delicious mixture of tuna and crunchy vegetables tucked into rolled, crisp lettuce leaves for a superlight lunch.

🕐 10 minutes   ◔ 2

- 1½ tbsp low-fat natural bio yogurt
- 85g/3oz canned tuna chunks in spring water, drained
- 50g/2oz cooked and cooled rice
- 85g/3oz frozen peas, cooked then refreshed in cold water
- ½ red pepper, deseeded and chopped
- 1 avocado, stoned, peeled and cut into chunks
- zest and juice 1 lime
- small pack coriander, leaves chopped
- 1 large Little Gem lettuce, or other crisp lettuce, such as cos

1 Combine all the ingredients except the lettuce in a bowl, season, then chill until ready to eat.
2 Spoon the tuna mix on top of the lettuce leaves, wrap up and enjoy.

PER SERVING 277 kcals, protein 20g, carbs 22g, fat 12g, sat fat 3g, fibre 8g, sugar 7g, salt 0.2g

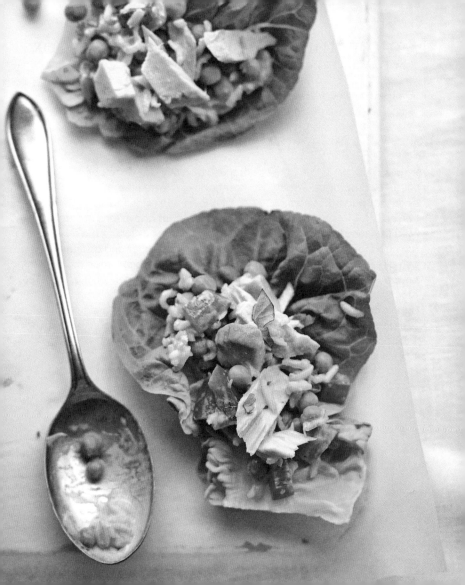

Lemony tuna & asparagus salad box

This high-protein lunch is surprisingly light in calories, so if you are looking for a good-looking starter to serve friends for supper, this is a winner.

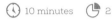 10 minutes 2

- 2 eggs
- 200g/7oz asparagus, woody ends snapped off, spears halved
- 160g can tuna in spring water (no need to drain)
- 1 small red onion, very finely chopped
- 125g/4½oz canned cannellini beans, drained and rinsed
- zest and juice ½ lemon
- 1 tbsp chopped dill
- 1 tsp extra virgin olive oil

1 Put a pan of water on to boil with a steamer set above it. When the water comes to the boil, lower the eggs into the water and steam the asparagus above for 8 minutes.

2 Meanwhile, gently toss all the other ingredients together and arrange on plates or in rigid containers. Plunge the eggs into cold water to cool them a little, then peel and quarter them.

3 Serve the eggs with the asparagus, tuna and bean salad. This will keep in the fridge for 2 days.

PER SERVING 279 kcals, protein 33g, carbs 12g, fat 10g, sat fat 2g, fibre 7g, sugar 4g, salt 1g

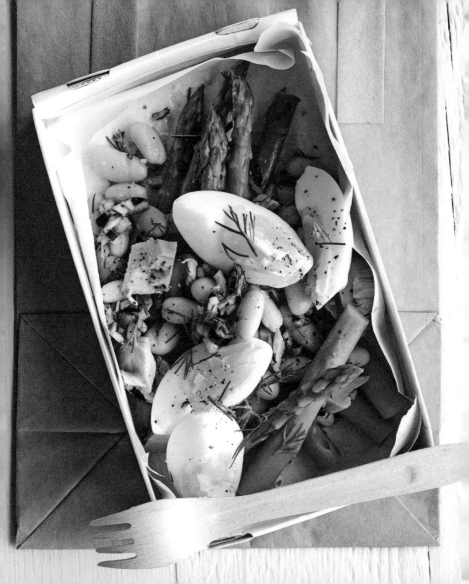

Mushroom & basil omelette with grilled tomatoes

An easy vegetarian lunch or brunch for two to share. Serve the omelette and tomatoes on their own or with a crisp green salad.

🕐 20 minutes 🥧 2

- 2 tomatoes, halved
- 3 medium eggs
- 1 tbsp snipped chives
- 1 tsp unsalted butter
- 300g/10oz chestnut mushrooms, sliced
- 2 tbsp low-fat soft cheese
- 1 tbsp finely torn basil leaves
- green salad, to serve (optional)

1 Heat grill to high and grill the tomatoes, turning occasionally to prevent burning, until slightly scorched. Keep warm.

2 Beat the eggs in a bowl, add a small splash of water and mix. Add the chives and some black pepper, and beat again. Set aside.

3 In a non-stick frying pan, heat the butter over a medium heat until foaming. Cook the mushrooms for 5–8 minutes until tender, stirring occasionally. Remove and set aside.

4 Briskly stir the egg mixture, then add to the hot pan (tilting it so that the mixture covers the entire base). Leave for 10 seconds or so until it begins to set then gently stir to cook any unset egg.

5 Spoon the mushroom mix to one side of the omelette and top with the cheese and basil. Flip the omelette, if you like. Cook for 1 minute more, cut in half and slide on to plates. Serve with the tomatoes and a green salad, if you like.

PER SERVING 196 kcals, protein 14g, carbs 4g, fat 14g, sat fat 5g, fibre 3g, sugar 4g, salt 0.5g

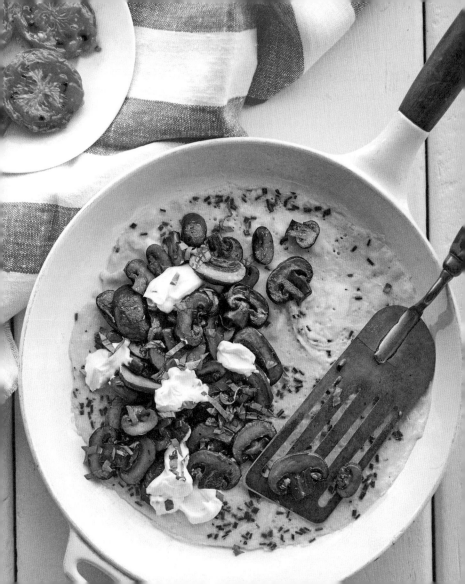

Asparagus salad with a runny poached egg

A simple, balanced bistro-style salad that's low in calories but high in flavour, texture and nutrition.

🕐 13 minutes   ◖ 2

- 1 tbsp extra virgin olive oil
- 1 tbsp balsamic vinegar
- 200g/7oz peeled cooked beetroot (not in vinegar), cut into bite-sized pieces
- 2 handfuls mixed salad leaves
- ¼ cucumber, cut into batons
- 8 asparagus spears, trimmed
- 2 eggs

1 Pour the olive oil and vinegar into a small bowl, mix well to make a dressing and add the beetroot. Divide the mixed leaves and cucumber between two plates.

2 Blanch the asparagus in a pan of simmering water for 2 minutes, then remove to a plate. Crack the eggs into the pan and simmer gently for 3 minutes until the whites are cooked and the yolks are just beginning to set, but still runny. Remove the eggs with a slotted spoon and drain on kitchen paper.

3 Meanwhile, add the beetroot to the salad plates, pour over the dressing and lightly toss together. Top each plate with the asparagus and a poached egg to serve.

PER SERVING 228 kcals, protein 13g, carbs 13g, fat 13g, sat fat 3g, fibre 5g, sugar 12g, salt 0.5g

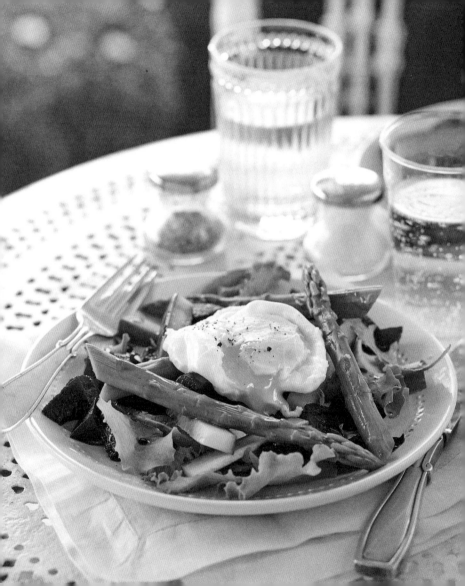

Courgette tortilla with toppings

This is a bit like an omelette pizza. The houmous goes well with egg, and red pepper makes a tasty, colourful contrast. Use leftover pepper in salads, dips or sandwiches.

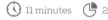 11 minutes 2

- 1 tbsp olive or rapeseed oil
- 1 large courgette, coarsely grated
- 1 tsp harissa paste
- 4 eggs
- 3 tbsp reduced-fat houmous
- 1 large red pepper from a jar (not in oil), torn into strips
- 3 pitted queen olives, quartered
- handful chopped coriander leaves

1 Heat the oil in a 20cm non-stick frying pan then add the courgette and cook for a few minutes, stirring occasionally, until softened. Meanwhile, beat the harissa with the eggs in a small bowl.

2 Pour the eggs into the pan and cook gently, stirring to allow the uncooked egg to flow through to the base of the pan. When it is two-thirds cooked, leave the tortilla untouched to set then slide on to a plate. Now return the tortilla to the pan uncooked-side down, to complete cooking.

3 To serve, tip the tortilla on to a board and spread with the houmous. Scatter with the pepper, olives and coriander. Cut in wedges and eat warm or cold.

PER SERVING 302 kcals, protein 18g, carbs 8g, fat 22g, sat fat 5g, fibre 2g, sugar 2g, salt 0.8g

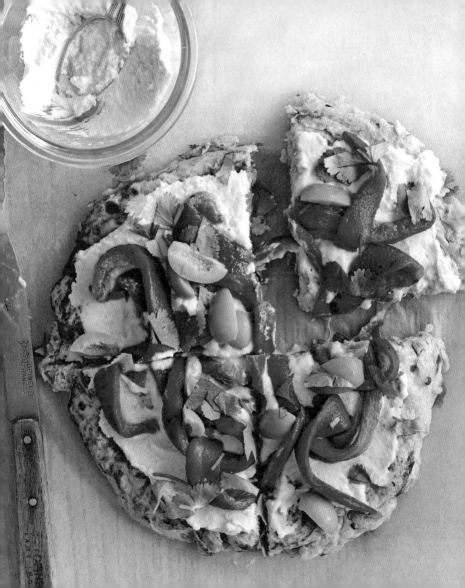

Egg & veggie pittas

Cram wholemeal bread pockets with healthy aubergine, beetroot and carrot, then add a garlic-and-dill yogurt and sliced hard-boiled eggs.

🕐 35 minutes   🥧 2

- 1 aubergine, cut into thick rounds
- 1½ tbsp olive or rapeseed oil
- 1 tbsp harissa paste
- 2 eggs
- 1 tbsp red wine vinegar
- 2 tsp agave nectar or clear honey
- 1 raw beetroot, grated
- 1 large carrot, peeled and julienned
- ½ small red onion, very finely sliced
- 4 tbsp 0%-fat Greek yogurt
- 1 tbsp chopped dill fronds
- 1 garlic clove, crushed
- 2 wholemeal pitta breads

1 Heat oven to 220C/200C fan/gas 7. Put the aubergine slices on a baking sheet, season, brush with oil and bake for 15 minutes. Turn the aubergine slices, spread them with the harissa and bake for another 5 minutes.

2 Meanwhile, carefully lower the eggs into a pan of boiling water, turn down the heat and simmer for 10 minutes. Run the eggs under cold water to cool, peel and put to one side.

3 In a bowl, mix the vinegar and agave or honey with some seasoning, then tip in the beetroot, carrot and onion. In another bowl, mix together the yogurt, dill, garlic and some seasoning.

4 Toast the pittas and split them in half. Slice the eggs and put them inside the pittas with the spicy aubergine rounds and some of the beetroot salad. Spoon in some of the yogurt and serve with the remaining aubergine and the rest of the salad and yogurt on the side.

PER SERVING 387 kcals, protein 20g, carbs 41g, fat 16g, sat fat 3g, fibre 9g, sugar 15g, salt 0.8g

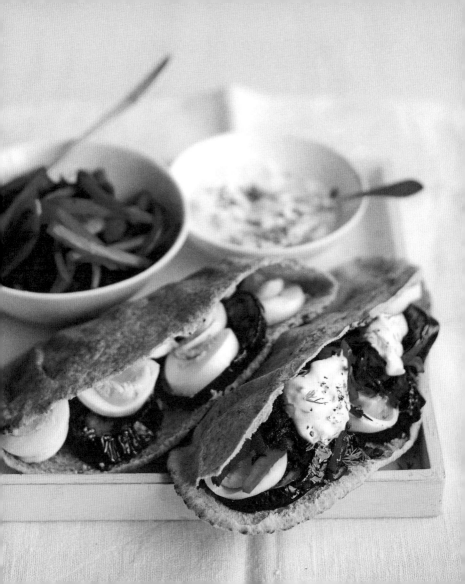

Curried egg-mayo open sandwich

When you're having a hectic day a sandwich is a quick option for a light lunch. Use one slice of bread, then pile on the filling with salad to make it more substantial.

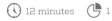 12 minutes 🥧 1

- a little curry paste
- 1 tbsp low-fat mayonnaise
- small squirt tomato purée
- 1 boiled egg, shelled and chopped
- 1 slice rye bread or seeded wholemeal
- several Little Gem lettuce leaves
- 1 spring onion, chopped
- few slices cucumber

1 Mix the curry paste with the mayo and tomato purée then stir in the egg. Pile the mixture onto the bread with the lettuce, spring onion and cucumber.

PER SERVING 196 kcals, protein 14g, carbs 41g, fat 18g, sat fat 3g, fibre 8g, sugar 7g, salt 1.5g

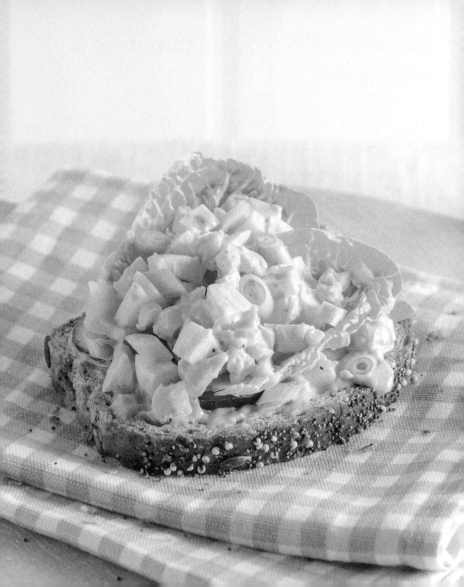

Tartines with roasted tomatoes & mint pesto

· ·

French open-faced cheese-and-tomato toasts, spread with ricotta and drizzled with a light mint-and-garlic pesto. A delicious treat you can easily make more of for friends.

🕐 30 minutes   🍽 2

- 4 medium-sized vine-ripened tomatoes, halved
- 2 tbsp extra virgin olive oil
- 2 thick slices wholemeal bread
- 1 garlic clove, left whole
- 15g/½oz pine nuts, toasted
- ½ small bunch mint
- ½ tbsp balsamic vinegar
- 50g/2oz ricotta
- green salad, to serve (optional)

1 Heat oven to 190C/170C fan/gas 5. Put the tomato halves in a roasting tin in a single layer. Drizzle with 1 tablespoon of the oil, season well and roast for 20 minutes. Set aside.

2 Toast the bread, then rub with the garlic – save the clove for the pesto. Brush a bit more of the oil over the toast and put on two plates.

3 Using a food processor, whizz together the pine nuts, mint, garlic, remaining oil and the vinegar to make a pesto. Thickly spread the ricotta on the toast, then top with the roasted tomatoes and drizzles of the mint pesto. Serve with a green salad, if you like.

· ·

PER SERVING 333 kcals, protein 10g, carbs 28g, fat 20g, sat fat 4g, fibre 5g, sugar 8g, salt 0.8g

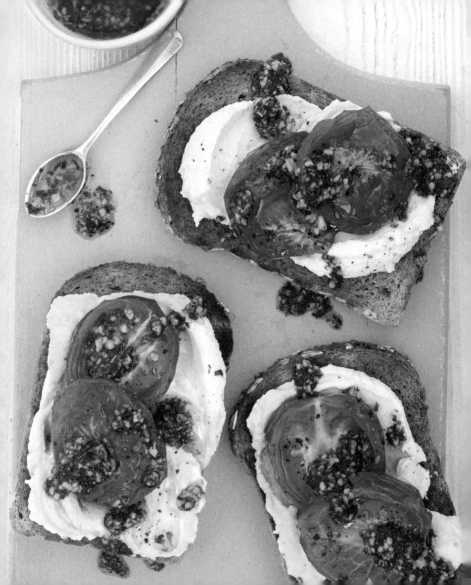

Houmous & avocado pitta

Fast, filling and really speedy for when you are hungry and in a hurry, especially if you use the toaster to warm the pitta.

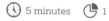 5 minutes 1

- 1 wholemeal pitta, warmed rather than toasted
- 2 spoonfuls houmous, low-fat if you like
- ½ small avocado, diced
- squeeze lemon, plus extra wedges to serve
- ½ small red onion, chopped
- few coriander leaves
- 2–3 cherry tomatoes, halved
- 1 small roasted red pepper from a jar (not in oil), optional, chopped

1 Cut the pitta in half then stuff a spoonful of houmous in each piece. Add the avocado tossed with the lemon juice, along with the red onion, coriander, tomatoes and roasted pepper, if using. Squeeze in extra lemon if you like and eat while still warm.

PER SERVING 364 kcals, protein 14g, carbs 41g, fat 18g, sat fat 3g, fibre 8g, sugar 7g, salt 1.5g

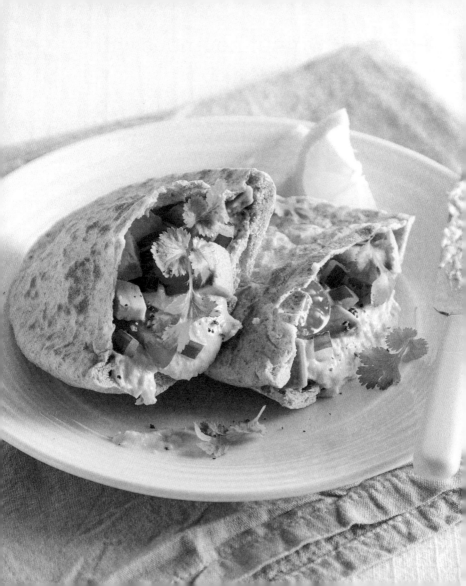

Pepper & walnut houmous with veggie dippers

· · · · · · · · · · · · · · · · · · · ·

Pack in the veg with this quick-to-make chickpea, sesame and walnut dip blitzed with roasted sweet red pepper.

🕐 10 minutes   🍽 2

- 400g can chickpeas, drained and rinsed
- 1 garlic clove
- 1 large roasted red pepper from a jar (not in oil), about 100g/4oz
- 1 tbsp tahini (sesame paste)
- juice ½ lemon
- 4 walnut halves, chopped
- 2 courgettes, 2 carrots, 2 celery sticks, all cut into fingers

1 Tip the chickpeas, garlic, pepper, tahini and lemon juice into a bowl to make the houmous and blitz with a hand blender or in a food processor to a thick purée. Stir in the walnuts.

2 Pack the houmous into pots and serve with the veggie dippers. Will keep in the fridge for 2 days, although the veg are best prepared fresh to preserve their vitamins.

· ·

PER SERVING 296 kcals, protein 14g, carbs 30g, fat 13g, sat fat 2g, fibre 12g, sugar 9g, salt 0.8g

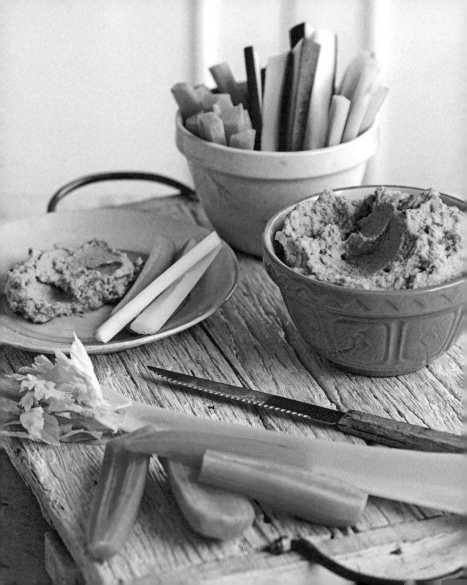

Chickpea patties with carrot & raisin salad

. . . .

If taking this salad to work, don't dress it in the morning with the oil and vinegar as the salad will wilt, take a wedge of lemon instead and squeeze it over just before eating.

🕐 16 minutes   🥧 2

- 400g can chickpeas, drained and rinsed
- 1 garlic clove, chopped
- 1 egg
- 1 tbsp ground almonds
- 2 tsp harissa paste
- 1 tsp ground cumin
- 3 tbsp chopped parsley leaves
- 2 tsp rapeseed oil, for frying

FOR THE SALAD & DRESSING

- 1 carrot and 1 courgette, shaved into strips with a peeler
- 5 radishes thinly sliced
- 2 handfuls watercress, rocket and spinach salad leaves
- 1 tbsp raisins
- 1 tsp each white wine vinegar and flaxseed or rapeseed oil

1 Tip the chickpeas, garlic, egg, almonds, harissa and cumin into a bowl, and blitz with a hand blender until smooth. Stir in the parsley.

2 Heat the oil in a non-stick frying pan. Dollop the chickpea mixture into the pan in 4 big spoonfuls, spaced apart, and cook for 3 minutes each side.

3 Toss the veg leaves and raisins together for the salad, but don't dress with the oil and vinegar until you are about to eat the salad with the patties.

. . . .

PER SERVING 316 kcals, protein 17g, carbs 31g, fat 14g, sat fat 2g, fibre 9g, sugar 12g, salt 1g

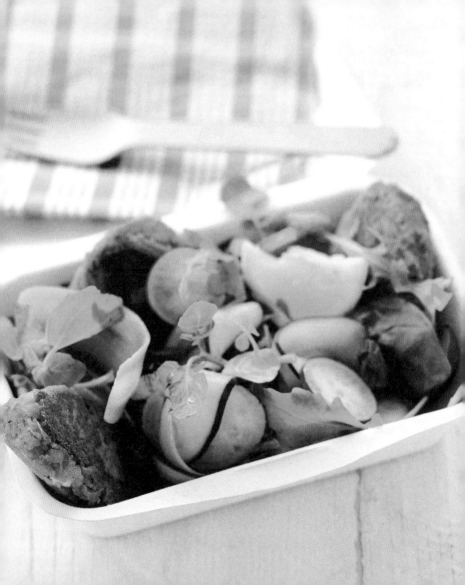

Asparagus soup

· ·

A super green and super tasty soup made from just a few simple ingredients. This recipe serves 4, but any leftovers will keep in the fridge for a couple of days.

🕐 30 minutes   🥘 4

- 15g/½oz butter
- 1 tbsp rapeseed oil
- 350g/12oz asparagus spears, stalks chopped, woody ends discarded, tips reserved
- 3 shallots, finely sliced
- 2 garlic cloves, crushed
- 2 large handfuls spinach leaves
- 700ml/1¼ pints vegetable stock (fresh, if possible)
- olive oil, for drizzling (optional)
- rustic bread (preferably sourdough), to serve (optional)

1 Heat the butter and oil in a large pan until foaming. Fry the asparagus tips for a few minutes to soften. Remove and set aside.

2 Add the shallots, asparagus stalks and garlic to the pan, and cook for 5–10 minutes until softened but still bright. Stir through the spinach, pour over the stock, bring to the boil then blitz with a hand blender.

3 Season the soup generously and add hot water to loosen, if needed. Ladle the soup into bowls and scatter the asparagus tips over each. Drizzle with olive oil and serve with sourdough bread, if you like.

· ·

PER SERVING 102 kcals, protein 4g, carbs 4g, fat 7g, sat fat 2g, fibre 4g, sugar 4g, salt 0.6g

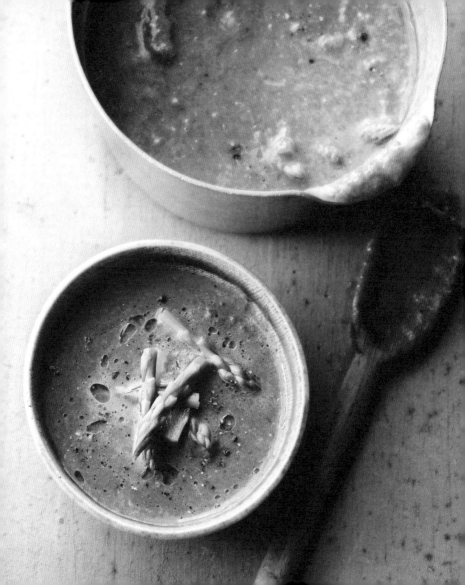

Moroccan-roasted-veg soup

Roasted roots are perfect for soup – this recipe uses parsnips and carrots with butternut squash and is flavoured with ras-el-hanout spice mix.

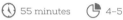 55 minutes 4–5

- 1 red onion, cut into 8 wedges
- 300g/10oz carrots, cut into 2cm/¾in chunks
- 300g/10oz parsnips, cut into 2cm/¾in chunks
- 300g/10oz peeled butternut squash, deseeded and cut into 2cm/¾in chunks
- 1 small potato, cut into 2cm/¾in chunks
- 2 garlic cloves
- 1 tbsp ras-el-hanout spice mix
- 1½ tbsp rapeseed or olive oil
- 1.3 litres/2¼ pints hot vegetable stock
- dollops of Greek-style yogurt and 1 tbsp finely chopped mint leaves, to garnish (optional)

1 Heat oven to 200C/180C fan/gas 6. Tip all the vegetables and the garlic into a roasting tin. Sprinkle over the ras-el-hanout spice mix and some seasoning, drizzle over the oil and give everything a good stir. Roast for 30–35 minutes, turning the vegetables over halfway, until they're tender and starting to caramelise a little.

2 Transfer the roasted veg to a large pan, pour over the hot stock and simmer for 5 minutes. Purée the soup in a food processor, or in the pan with a hand blender, until smooth, then ladle into a flask for work. If eating at home, serve with a dollop of yogurt, a scattering of chopped mint and a grinding of black pepper.

PER SERVING (5) 187 kcals, protein 5g, carbs 29g, fat 6g, sat fat 1g, fibre 10g, sugar 17g, salt 0.9g

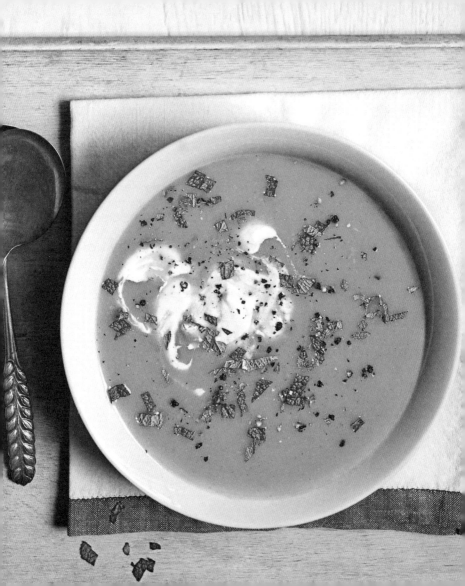

Fattoush

• •

This classic Middle Eastern salad makes a crunchy, light side dish or lunchbox filler –
it's sprinkled with sumac, the tangy Middle-Eastern spice, mint and parsley.

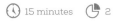 15 minutes   2

FOR THE SALAD
- 2 tomatoes, chopped into chunks
- ¼ cucumber, deseeded and sliced
- ½ red onion, sliced
- 1 small head romaine lettuce, shredded
- handful mint leaves, roughly chopped
- handful parsley leaves, roughly chopped
- 1 tsp sumac
- 2 pitta breads

FOR THE DRESSING
- ½ garlic clove, crushed
- 2 tbsp red wine vinegar
- 1 tbsp extra virgin olive oil
- juice ½ lemon

1 The night before, toss together all the salad ingredients except for the pitta bread and sumac. Make up the dressing and season to taste. Leave these separate until the morning

2 The next morning, arrange the salad on a large platter, or in boxes for a picnic, and sprinkle over the sumac. Toast the pitta breads until lightly golden and when cool, tear into pieces and combine with the salad and dressing.

• •
PER SERVING 358 kcals, protein 12g, carbs 57g, fat 18g, sat fat 1g, fibre 6g, sugar 10g, salt 1.1g

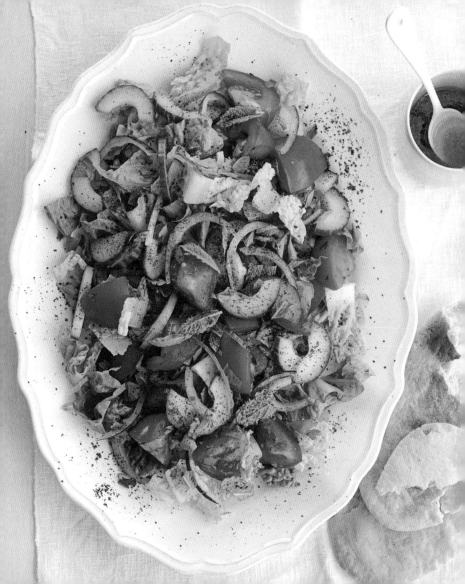

Mini spinach & cottage-cheese frittatas

Tiny omelette bites that are ideal for lunchboxes – dill, nutmeg and spring onion keep them flavour-packed. Serve two frittata per person with a little salad on the side.

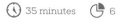 35 minutes   6

- butter, for greasing
- 85g/3oz baby leaf spinach
- 3 eggs
- 6 tbsp low-fat cottage cheese
- 3 spring onions, sliced
- few sprigs dill, roughly chopped
- generous grating nutmeg

1 Heat oven to 180C/160C fan/gas 4. Lightly grease a 6-hole muffin tin and line with squares of baking parchment to act as muffin cases (greasing the tin first will help to hold the parchment in place).

2 Put the spinach in a colander in the sink and pour over a kettle of boiling water, then leave to drain. When cool enough to handle, squeeze as much liquid as you can from the spinach, then roughly chop.

3 Beat the eggs and season well. Marble through the spinach, cottage cheese, spring onions, dill and a generous grating of nutmeg. Divide the mixture among the muffin cases. Bake for 18–20 minutes or until just set. Leave to cool a little before removing from the tin. The frittatas will keep in an airtight container in the fridge for up to 3 days.

PER FRITTATA 59 kcals, protein 6g, carbs 1g, fat 3g, sat fat 1g, fibre none, sugar 1g, salt 0.3g

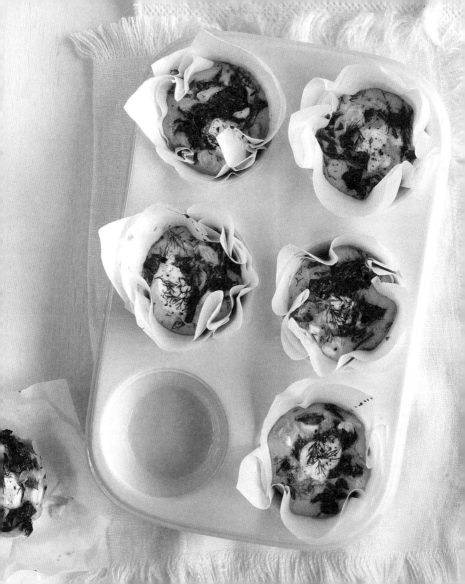

Cajun grilled chicken with lime, black-eyed bean salad & guacamole

· ·

Spice up your chicken with cayenne, oregano, paprika and thyme then serve on a salsa-like salad with an avocado dip. This makes enough for lunch the next day, too.

🕐 25 minutes   📊 2

FOR THE CHICKEN
- 1 tsp rapeseed oil
- 1 tsp smoked or regular paprika
- ¼ tsp cayenne pepper
- 1 garlic clove, finely chopped
- 2 boneless skinless chicken breasts, bashed to flatten

FOR THE SALAD & GUACAMOLE
- 200g/7oz canned black eye beans, drained and rinsed
- 2 tomatoes, diced
- 85g/3oz canned sweetcorn
- 2 spring onions, finely chopped
- 25g/1oz semi-dried tomatoes in oil from a jar, roughly chopped
- zest 1 lime and juice 2
- 2 handfuls coriander, chopped
- 1 small avocado
- ¼ red chilli, deseeded and finely chopped
- ½ tbsp olive oil

1 Mix together the oil, spices and garlic in a large sealable bag. Add the chicken and set aside to marinate for at least 15 minutes.

2 In a large bowl, mix the first five ingredients for the bean salad, adding half the coriander and the zest and juice of 1 lime. Stir well and set aside.

3 For the guacamole, scoop the flesh from the avocado and put it in a medium bowl, chopping it roughly with the side of the spoon. Add the chilli, oil, remaining lime juice and coriander, and mix well.

4 Heat grill to high. Line a grill pan with foil, and grill the chicken breasts for 5 minutes, checking occasionally. Once golden brown, turn and grill for a further 5–7 minutes. Check the middle of the breasts after 5 minutes and, if cooked through, remove from the heat. Put a warm chicken breast on each plate, with some bean salad and a dollop of guacamole on the side.

· ·

PER SERVING 491 kcals, protein 48g, carbs 30g, fat 20g, sat fat 4g, fibre 12g, sugar 10g, salt 1g

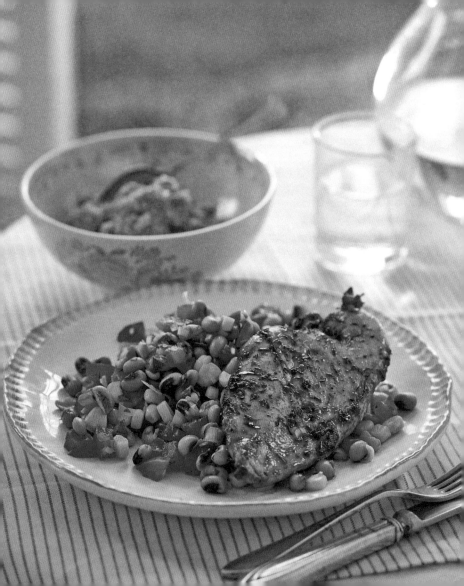

Lemon & garlic roast chicken with charred broccoli & sweet-potato mash

. . . .

A healthy all-in-one roast that supplies two portions of veg and a vitamin-C boost. Keep the rest of the chicken in the fridge for healthy lunches for the rest of the week.

🕐 1 hour 10 minutes – 1 hour 25 minutes   🥧 2

- 1 small free-range chicken (about 1kg/ 2lb 4oz)
- 2 garlic cloves, halved
- 1 tsp rapeseed oil
- small bunch thyme
- 1 lemon, halved
- 1 small head broccoli (about 200g/7oz), cut into small florets
- 200g/7oz sweet potatoes, peeled and cubed
- 1 tbsp low-fat soft cheese

1 Heat oven to 200C/180C fan/gas 6. Put the chicken in a large roasting tin and rub it with 1 garlic half. Drizzle with oil, then stuff the cavity with thyme, 1 lemon half and the garlic just used. Cut the other lemon half in two and put in the tin with the garlic.

2 Cover with foil and roast for 40 minutes, then remove the foil and spoon over the hot juices. Arrange the broccoli in the tin and cook for 20–30 minutes. To check the chicken is cooked, pierce the thigh – the juices should run clear. Re-cover with foil and set aside.

3 Put the potatoes in a pan of boiling water and simmer for 7–10 minutes until tender. Drain, and mash with the soft cheese.

4 Divide the broccoli between two plates. Transfer the chicken to a serving plate and discard the lemon and garlic. Skim the fat from the juices and pour the liquid into a jug.

5 Carve the chicken, serving 2 slices per person along with the veg. Drizzle over the juices.

. . . .

PER SERVING 369 kcals, protein 34g, carbs 32g, fat 12g, sat fat 4g, fibre 8g, sugar 16g, salt 0.5g

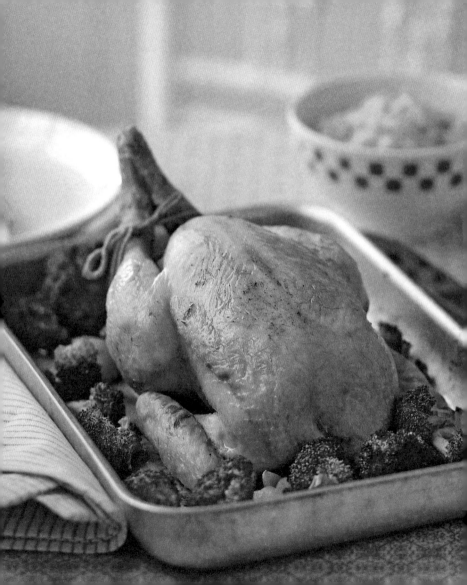

Easy one-pot chicken casserole

Make this in the evening, eat one portion then freeze the rest for a tasty meal another day when you are too tired to cook.

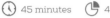 45 minutes 4

- 8 bone-in chicken thighs, skin removed
- 1 tbsp olive or rapeseed oil
- 5 spring onions, sliced
- 2 tbsp plain flour
- 2 chicken stock cubes, preferably reduced-salt
- 2 carrots, cut into batons
- 400g/14oz new potatoes, halved if large
- 200g/7oz frozen peas
- 1 tbsp grainy mustard
- small handful soft herbs, such as chives, parsley, tarragon, leaves snipped/chopped

1 Put the kettle on. Fry the thighs in the oil in a casserole or wide pan with a lid quickly to brown. Stir in the whites of the spring onion with the flour and crumbled stock cubes until the flour disappears, then gradually stir in 750ml/1¼ pint hot water from the kettle. Throw in the carrots and potatoes; bring to a simmer. Cover and cook for 20 minutes.

2 Take off the lid and simmer the chicken and veg for 15 minutes more, then throw in the peas for another 5 minutes. Season, stir in the mustard, green spring-onion bits, the herbs and some seasoning.

PER SERVING 386 kcals, protein 42g, carbs 32g, fat 9g, sat fat 2g, fibre 6g, sugar 7g, salt 2.1g

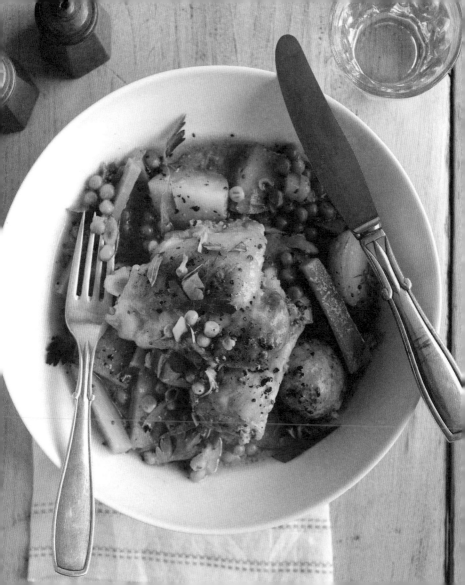

Chicken & pomegranate bulghar pilaf

Although this serves four, the recipe will easily halve. However, keep what is left in the fridge and it will make a tasty lunch the next day.

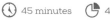 45 minutes 4

- a little rapeseed oil, for frying
- 8 chicken skinless thigh fillets
- 2 tbsp ras-el-hanout or Moroccan tagine spice mix
- 500ml/18 floz hot chicken stock, preferably reduced-salt
- 350g/12oz bulghar wheat
- bunch mint, chopped, plus a few leaves, to garnish
- 2 x 100g tubs pomegranate seeds

1 Heat a little oil in a large casserole dish (with a tight-fitting lid). Coat the chicken pieces with some seasoning and half of the spice mix and add to the pan; brown well on all sides.

2 Add the remaining spice mix and cook for 1 minute. Pour over the stock, season and stir, then cover and cook for 25 minutes over a low–medium heat.

3 Remove the lid, increase the heat to a medium simmer and add the bulghar wheat. Cook for 10 minutes, then re-cover, turn off the heat and leave to stand for a further 10 minutes.

4 When all the liquid has been absorbed and the bulghar wheat is tender, stir through the chopped mint and scatter over the pomegranate seeds and a few mint leaves to serve.

PER SERVING 369 kcals, protein 34g, carbs 32g, fat 12g, sat fat 4g, fibre 8g, sugar 16g, salt 0.5g

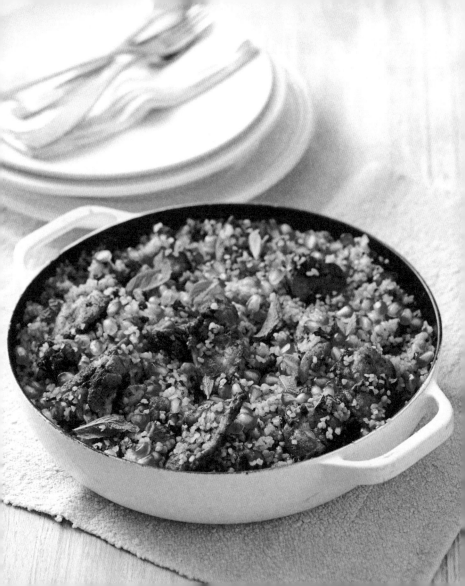

Chicken & lentil stew with gremolata

Spruce up a light tomato-based casserole with a generous sprinkling of parsley, lemon and garlic – also known as 'gremolata'. Perfect for entertaining.

 1 hour 5 minutes   4

- 2 tbsp olive or rapeseed oil
- 8 chicken drumsticks
- 2 onions, very finely chopped
- 6 tbsp red split lentils
- 400g can chopped tomatoes
- 1 chicken stock cube, preferably reduced-salt, crumbled

FOR THE GREMOLATA

- zest 1 lemon
- 1 garlic clove, finely chopped
- small handful parsley leaves, finely chopped

1 Heat half the oil in a large flameproof casserole dish, brown the drumsticks on all sides, then transfer to a plate.

2 Add the onions and remaining oil to the pan, and cook for 5 minutes or so until soft. Add the lentils, tomatoes, 1 can water and the stock cube. Return the drumsticks to the pan. Bring to the boil, then turn down the heat, put on a lid and simmer for 30 minutes or until tender. Keep an eye on the stew and add a little water if it is drying out. Remove the lid and cook for another 10 minutes, or until the sauce has thickened, then season.

3 Meanwhile, make the gremolata. Mix the lemon zest, garlic and parsley together and sprinkle over the cooked stew to serve.

PER SERVING 337 kcals, protein 32g, carbs 20g, fat 15g, sat fat 3g, fibre 4g, sugar 7g, salt 1.2g

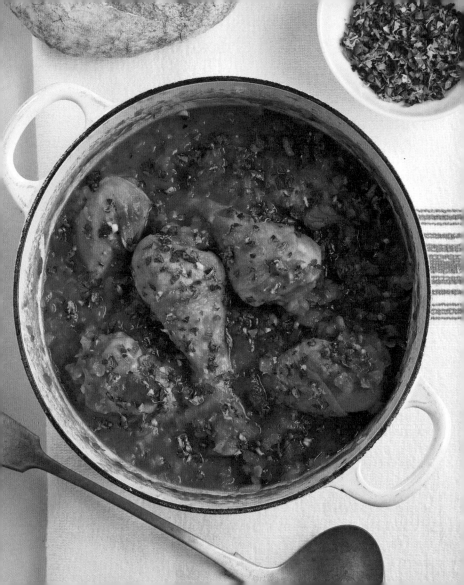

Fragrant spiced chicken with banana sambal

· ·

This makes six portions so freeze what you don't eat. The sambal and rice serve two, so double or triple to adjust for more servings.

🕐 1 hour   🕒 6

- 2 large onions, quartered
- 4 garlic cloves
- thumb-size piece ginger
- 600ml/1 pint chicken stock
- 1 tsp each ground coriander and cumin
- ½ tsp ground turmeric
- 4 green cardamom pods
- 1 large red chilli, deseeded and finely chopped
- 2 tbsp ground almonds
- 2 tbsp tomato purée
- 500g/1lb 2oz skinless chicken breasts, cubed
- small pack coriander, chopped

FOR THE SAMBAL & RICE (FOR 2)
- ½ red onion, finely chopped
- ¼ cucumber, diced
- 1 small banana, diced
- zest and juice ½ lime
- 250g pack ready-cooked brown basmati rice

1 Put the onions in a food processor with the garlic and ginger. Blitz until it is as smooth as it will go then pour in the stock and blitz again.

2 Heat a large non-stick pan, sprinkle in the spices and toast for a minute. Pour in the onion mixture with 300ml/½ pint water and all but ½ teaspoon of the chopped chilli; add the almonds and tomato purée, and stir well. Cover and simmer for 35 minutes until the mixture is pulpy and the onions are completely cooked, stirring every now and then. Top up with water if the mixture is too thick before it is fully cooked.

3 Add the chicken and half the coriander, cover and cook very gently for a few minutes more to cook the chicken through. Mix all the sambal ingredients with the remaining fresh coriander and chilli. Serve the chicken and sambal with the brown rice, heated according to the pack instructions.

· ·

PER SERVING 410 kcals, protein 34g, carbs 48g, fat 9g, sat fat 2g, fibre 5g, sugar 15g, salt 1.2g

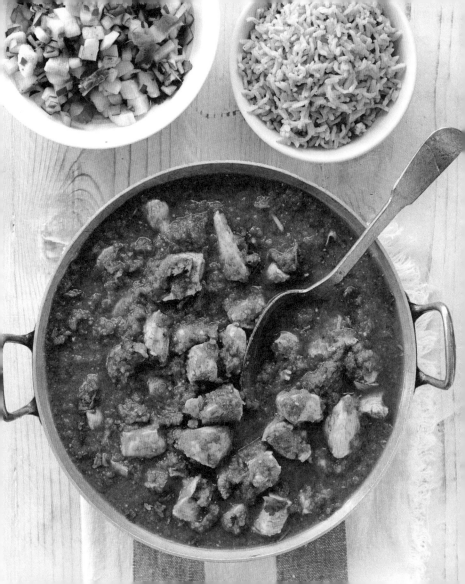

Baked peanut chicken with carrot & cucumber salad

. . . .

Some peanut butters contain added sugar, so try to find one without. Here it makes a tasty crust for skinless oven-baked chicken served with a refreshing salad.

🕐 30 minutes 🍽 2

FOR THE PEANUT CHICKEN

- 2 tbsp crunchy peanut butter, with no added sugar
- 1 garlic clove, finely grated
- ½ tsp each ground cumin, coriander and smoked paprika
- 1 medium egg
- 2 skinless chicken breast fillets

FOR THE SALAD & DRESSING

- 1 tbsp cider vinegar
- 1 tsp rapeseed oil
- 2 large handfuls salad leaves
- 10cm/4in piece cucumber, halved and sliced
- 1 carrot, coarsely grated
- 1 small banana shallot, halved and thinly sliced
- good handful chopped coriander leaves

1 Heat oven to 180C/160C fan/gas 4 and line a baking sheet with baking paper. Put the peanut butter, garlic, spices and egg in a small bowl, and whisk with a fork until blended. Add the chicken breasts one at a time, turning them in the mixture until completely coated then put on the baking sheet. Any remaining mix left in the bowl can be put on top of the chicken. Bake for 20 minutes until the coating is firm and the chicken is tender.

2 Mix the vinegar and oil for the dressing in a bowl then add the salad leaves, cucumber, carrot, shallot and coriander. Mix well and serve with the chicken.

. . . .
PER SERVING 321 kcals, protein 39g, carbs 7g, fat 14g, sat fat 3g, fibre 4g, sugar 6g, salt 0.5g

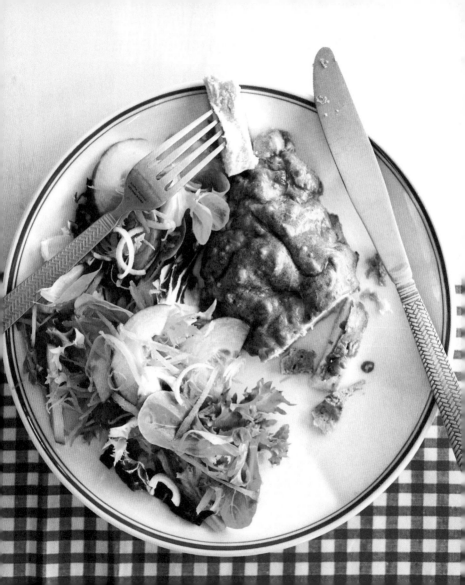

Chicken & cherry-tomato lentils

A simple but tasty traybake that combines storecupboard pulses with chicken thighs, cumin and parsley.

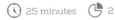 25 minutes 2

- 250g/9oz skinless chicken thigh fillets, cut into chunks
- 1 red onion, cut into wedges through the root
- 1 tbsp olive oil
- 100g/4oz cherry tomatoes
- ½ tbsp cumin seeds
- 250g pouch microwave Puy lentils
- 1 tbsp red wine vinegar
- small handful parsley leaves, chopped

1 Heat oven to 200C/180C fan/gas 6. Toss the chicken and onion with the oil, arrange in a roasting tin and season. Roast for 10 minutes, then add the cherry tomatoes and sprinkle over the cumin seeds. Cook for another 10 minutes.

2 Meanwhile, heat the Puy lentils according to the pack instructions. Once the chicken is ready, add the lentils to the tin and toss everything together. Stir in the red wine vinegar, parsley and seasoning to taste.

PER SERVING 356 kcals, protein 41g, carbs 31g, fat 9g, sat fat 2g, fibre 10g, sugar 5g, salt 1.7g

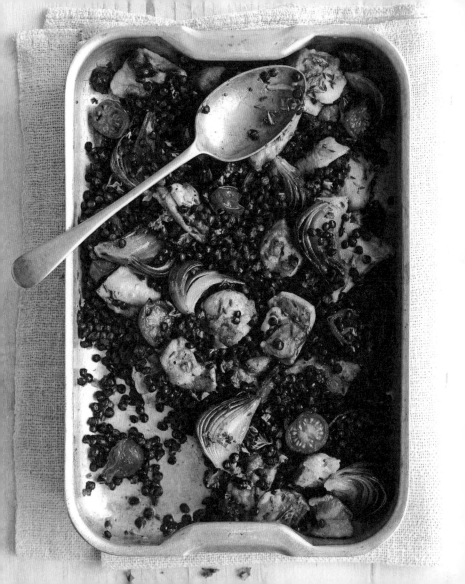

Tasty turkey meatballs

Oats, rather than breadcrumbs, give these meatballs a great texture while also having a lower GI. Ideal for feeding the family or freezing for another day.

🕐 45 minutes   🥧 4

FOR THE SAUCE
- 1 tbsp rapeseed oil, plus extra for frying
- 1 onion, finely chopped
- 2 carrots and 2 celery sticks, finely diced
- 2 garlic cloves, sliced thinly
- 1 fennel bulb, leaves reserved, halved and thinly sliced
- 500g carton tomato passata
- 500ml/18fl oz reduced-salt chicken stock
- 2 tbsp chopped parsley

FOR THE MEATBALLS
- 400g pack lean turkey breast mince
- 4 tbsp porridge oats
- 1 tsp fennel seeds, crushed
- 1 garlic clove, crushed

TO SERVE
- broccoli and baby new potatoes or pasta and salad

1 Heat the oil for the sauce in a large non-stick frying pan, with a lid, then tip in the onion, carrots, celery, garlic and sliced fennel, and stir well. Cover the pan and cook over a medium heat for 8 minutes, stirring every now and then. Pour in the passata and stock, cover and leave to simmer for 20 minutes.

2 Meanwhile, tip the mince for the meatballs into a large bowl, add the oats, fennel seeds and reserved leaves and the garlic with plenty of black pepper, and mix with your hands. Lightly shape into 25 meatballs about the size of a walnut. Spray or rub a non-stick pan with a little oil then gently cook the meatballs until they take on some colour. Give the sauce a stir then add the meatballs, cover and cook for 5 minutes until they are cooked through and the vegetables in the sauce are tender.

3 Serve scattered with the parsley accompanied by broccoli and baby new potatoes in their skins or pasta and salad.

PER SERVING 322 kcals, protein 38g, carbs 21g, fat 9g, sat fat 2g, fibre 7g, sugar 13g, salt 0.3g

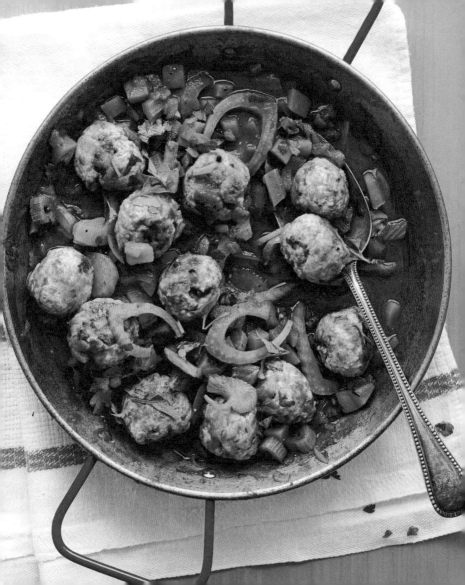

Prawn jalfrezi

. . . .

Three of your 5-a-day – onions, tomatoes and peppers – are packed into this lovely curry. The sauce also works with leftover cooked chicken or turkey instead of prawns.

🕐 30 minutes 🍽 2

- 2 tsp rapeseed oil
- 2 medium onions, chopped
- thumb-size piece ginger, finely chopped
- 2 garlic cloves, chopped
- 1 tsp ground coriander
- ½ tsp ground turmeric
- ½ tsp ground cumin
- ¼ tsp chilli flakes (or less if you don't like it too spicy)
- 400g can chopped tomatoes
- squeeze clear honey
- 1 large green pepper, halved, deseeded and chopped
- small bunch coriander, stalks and leaves separated, chopped
- 140g/5oz large cooked peeled tiger prawns
- 250g pouch cooked brown rice
- minty yogurt or mango chutney, to serve (optional)

1 Heat the oil in a non-stick pan and fry the onions, ginger and garlic for 8–10 minutes, stirring frequently, until softened and starting to colour. Add the spices and chilli flakes, stir briefly, then pour in the tomatoes with half a can of water and the honey.

2 Blitz everything in the pan with a hand blender until almost smooth (or use a food processor). Stir in the pepper and coriander stalks, cover the pan and leave to simmer for 10 minutes. (The mixture will be very thick and splutter a little, so stir frequently.)

3 Stir in the prawns and scatter over the coriander leaves. Heat the rice according to the pack instructions. Serve both with a minty yogurt or mango chutney, if you like.

. . . .

PER SERVING 335 kcals, protein 21g, carbs 48g, fat 7g, sat fat 1g, fibre 8g, sugar 15g, salt 1.5g

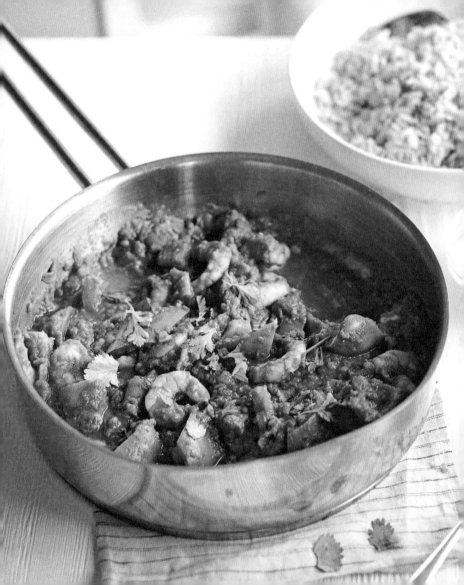

Salmon with salsa-verde new potatoes

Salsa verde is a punchy green sauce made from garlic, capers, basil, parsley, anchovies and lemon juice – the perfect foil for fish.

🕐 25 minutes   🥧 2, with leftover salsa verde

- 250g/9oz new potatoes, halved
- 2 salmon fillets, skin on (about 140g/5oz each)
- 3 tbsp olive oil
- 1 shallot, roughly chopped
- small bunch flat-leaf parsley, leaves roughly chopped
- small bunch basil, roughly torn
- 2 tbsp capers
- 4 anchovies, roughly chopped
- 1 large garlic clove, roughly chopped
- juice 1 lemon
- sugar snap peas, to serve (optional)

1 Put the potatoes in a pan of salted water, bring to the boil and cook for 15 minutes or until tender.

2 Heat a non-stick frying pan over a high heat and cook the salmon, skin-side down, for 10 minutes until the skin is crisp. Turn over and cook for another 4 minutes.

3 Put the oil, shallot, parsley, basil, capers, anchovies, garlic and lemon juice in a small blender, and whizz to a green sauce. Add seasoning to taste. Toss 2 tablespoons of the sauce with the potatoes and serve with the salmon and some sugar snap peas, if you like

PER SERVING 384 kcals, protein 31g, carbs 21g, fat 20g, sat fat 3g, fibre 2g, sugar 1g, salt 0.5g

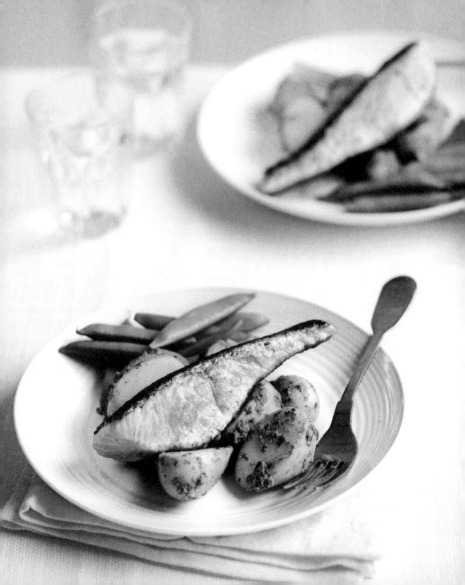

Toasted quinoa, lentil & poached-salmon salad

. . . .

Great if you're following a low-cholesterol diet, this plate of fresh greens contains nutty toasted supergrains and flavoursome lemon and herbs.

🕐 55 minutes 🍽 4

- 75g/2½oz quinoa
- 1 tsp olive oil
- 200ml/7fl oz light vegetable stock (we used Bouillon)
- 85g/3oz frozen soya beans
- 140g/5oz asparagus, trimmed
- 85g/3oz Tenderstem broccoli, florets trimmed and halved
- zest and juice 1 lemon
- 2 skinless salmon fillets (about 125g/5oz each)
- ½ garlic clove, crushed
- ½ x 250g pack ready-cooked Puy lentils
- 4 spring onions, sliced on the diagonal
- handful mint and parsley leaves, roughly chopped
- 50g/2oz baby leaf spinach
- 25g/1oz flaked almonds, toasted

1 Rinse the quinoa and tip into a non-stick frying pan over medium heat to dry the grains. Stir in the oil and cook, stirring, until the quinoa is a nutty brown and starts to 'pop'. Pour over the stock and simmer for 15–20 minutes until all the liquid has been absorbed. Tip into a bowl and allow to cool.

2 Meanwhile, bring a large pan of water to the boil. Simmer the soya beans, asparagus and broccoli for 2 minutes. Remove using a slotted spoon and plunge into ice-cold water. Drain.

3 Add 1 teaspoon of the lemon juice to the veg water in the pan and gently simmer. Season the salmon and poach for 6–8 minutes until just cooked. Remove, cool, then flake.

4 Combine the garlic, most of the lemon zest and the remaining juice. Combine with the quinoa, lentils, drained veg, spring onions, herbs and spinach in a large bowl, then season. Serve on plates, topped with salmon, the almonds and remaining lemon zest.

. . . .

PER SERVING 329 kcals, protein 26g, carbs 20g, fat 15g, sat fat 2g, fibre 6g, sugar 4g, salt 0.5g

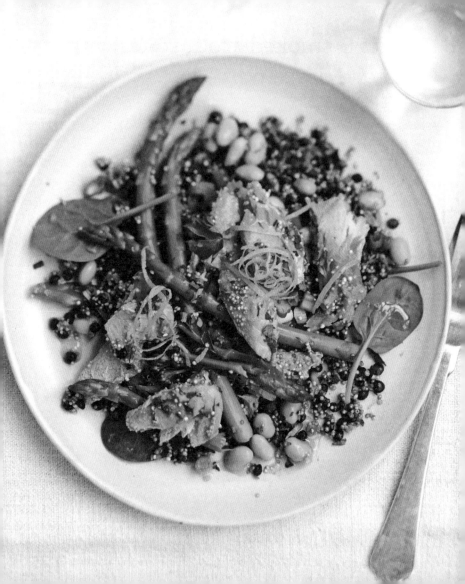

Potato & smoked-trout salad with mustard dressing

······················

A light smoked-fish salad with dill, capers and watercress in a tangy vinaigrette. Use mackerel instead of trout, if you like.

🕐 30 minutes   🍽 2

- 400g/14oz potatoes, unpeeled
- ½ tbsp red wine vinegar
- 1 tsp dill fronds, finely chopped
- ½ tbsp baby capers in brine, drained and rinsed
- ½ small red onion, thinly sliced into half moons
- handful watercress, leaves picked
- 85g/3oz skinless smoked trout (or mackerel) fillets, flesh broken into chunks

FOR THE DRESSING
- 1 tbsp wholegrain mustard
- 1 tbsp red wine vinegar
- 1 tbsp extra-virgin olive oil
- ½ tsp caster sugar

1 Put the potatoes in a pan of lightly salted water and bring to the boil. Simmer for 10 minutes or until tender, then drain. When cool enough to handle, peel and cut into thick slices. Put in a bowl and toss with the vinegar and some seasoning.

2 To make the dressing, mix all the ingredients together in a small bowl. Pour over the potatoes and add the dill, capers and onion. Arrange the potato salad on plates with the watercress, then top with the smoked fish.

···

PER SERVING 276 kcals, protein 14g, carbs 31g, fat 9g, sat fat 2g, fibre 5g, sugar 4g, salt 1.3g

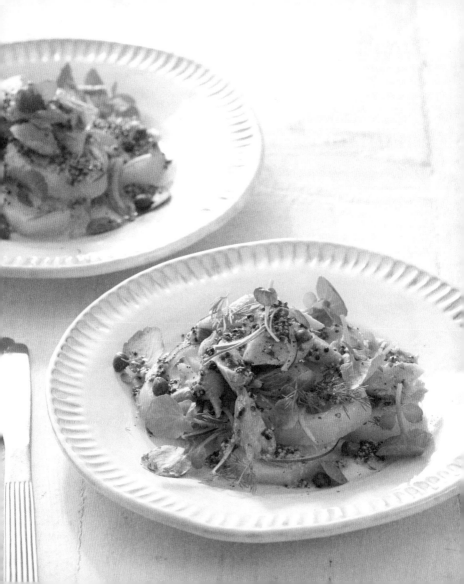

Simple herb-baked trout

A super simple whole baked fish with hot horseradish, zesty lemon and herbs – parsley, dill and thyme all work well – which is great on the taste buds and healthy too

🕐 25 minutes 🍽 2

- 2 whole rainbow trout, gutted and cleaned
- 1 tbsp olive or rapeseed oil
- 1 lemon, thinly sliced
- sprigs of your favourite herbs
- fresh horseradish, grated, to garnish (optional)
- your favourite seasonal veg, to serve

1 Heat oven to 220C/200C fan/gas 7. Lay the trout over a lightly oiled baking sheet and stuff the fish cavity with slices of lemon and the herbs. Season generously all over and drizzle with the remaining oil.

2 Bake in the oven for 20 minutes until the fish is cooked through – the eyes will have turned white and the flesh will be soft to touch. The trout can be served as they are with your favourite seasonal vegetables, but, for an added extra touch, peel away the top layer of skin and grate over fresh horseradish before serving.

PER SERVING 457 kcals, protein 63g, carbs 1g, fat 23g, sat fat 4g, fibre none, sugar 1g, salt 0.4g

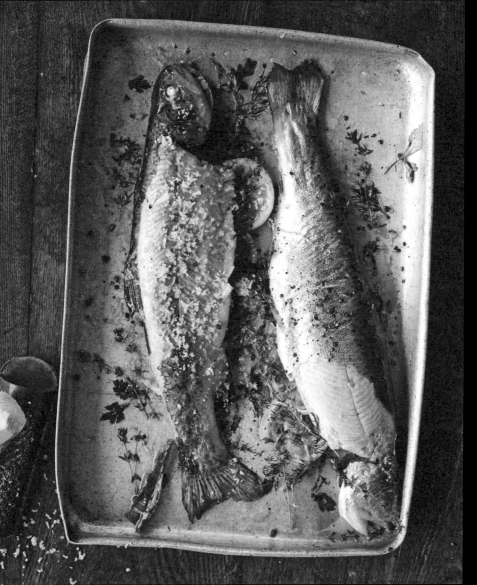

Fresh salmon trout with new potato & watercress salad

. . . .

Salmon trout is an oily fish that often gets overlooked in preference to salmon, but it is widely available. Try it in this warm salad of new potatoes, watercress and beans.

🕐 30 minutes   🥧 2

- 1 banana shallot, halved, ½ thinly sliced, ½ finely chopped
- 220g pack salmon trout fillets, skinned
- 1 tbsp chopped dill, plus 2 sprigs
- 1½ tbsp white wine vinegar
- 250g/9oz new potatoes, sliced
- 140g/5oz trimmed green beans, halved
- 1 tbsp extra virgin rapeseed oil
- 1 tsp wholegrain mustard
- 15g/½oz watercress, finely chopped

1 Heat oven to 200C/180C fan/gas 6. Take a square of foil and arrange the sliced shallot in the centre. Put the fish fillets on top, add the 2 dill sprigs and ½ tablespoon of the vinegar. Close the foil, sealing it to make a parcel, and put on a baking sheet. Put in the oven for 12 minutes once you start cooking the green beans in the next step.

2 Steam the potatoes for 6 minutes. Add the beans to the steamer then cook for 5 minutes more. Put the remaining vinegar in a large bowl with the oil, mustard, watercress and the chopped dill and shallot, and mix well. Add the warm beans and potatoes, and gently toss everything together. Serve with the fish, once cooked, pouring over the juices from the parcel.

. . . .

PER SERVING 378 kcals, protein 26g, carbs 24g, fat 19g, sat fat 3g, fibre 5g, sugar 3g, salt 0.3g

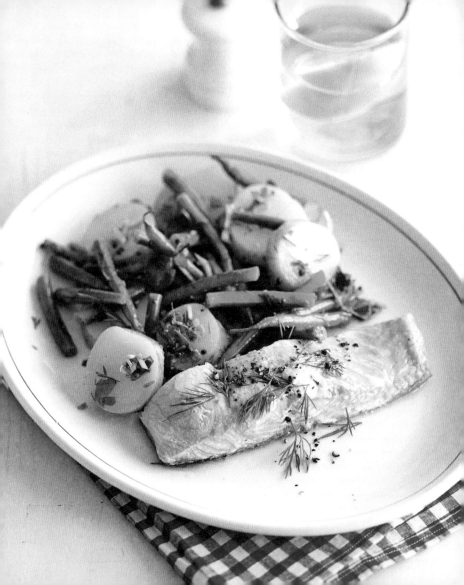

Salsa spaghetti with sardines

Canned sardines are a convenient source of oily fish, so they are well worth keeping in the store cupboard for a quick and easy supper like this.

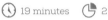 19 minutes   2

- 100g/4oz wholewheat spaghetti
- 2 large ripe tomatoes, finely chopped
- 1 red onion, very finely chopped
- 15g/½oz pitted Kalamata olives, quartered
- ½ tsp deseeded and finely chopped red chilli
- zest and juice ½ lemon, to taste
- 4 tbsp shredded basil leaves or 1 tsp chopped oregano leaves
- 2 x 120g cans sardines in olive oil, drained (oil reserved)

1 Cook the spaghetti according to the pack instructions. Meanwhile, mix the tomatoes with the onion, olives, chilli, lemon zest and basil or oregano. Heat the sardines in either the microwave or a pan.

2 Drain the pasta, return to the pan and toss well with the tomato mixture. Add the sardines in chunky pieces. Season with the lemon juice, some freshly ground black pepper, and a little of the reserved oil, if you like.

PER SERVING 442 kcals, protein 31g, carbs 43g, fat 16g, sat fat 3g, fibre 7g, sugar 10g, salt 1.7g

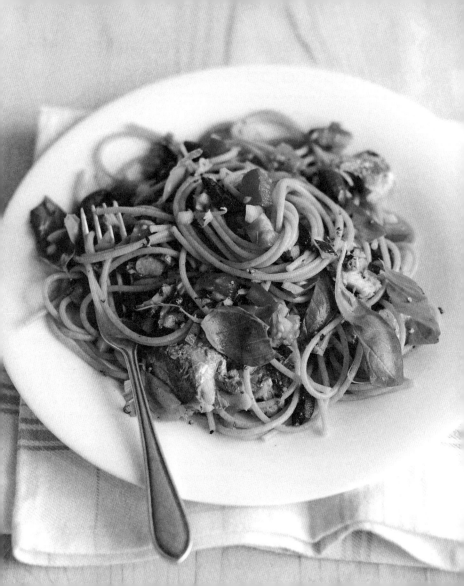

Grilled mackerel with orange, chilli & watercress salad
· ·

Mackerel is rich in omega-3 oils, but be careful of the total fat content. Oily mackerel and sardines are great with citrus and peppery leaves like rocket and watercress.

🕐 20 minutes 🥧 2

- ½ tsp black peppercorns
- ½ tsp coriander seeds
- 2 oranges
- 1 red chilli, deseeded and finely chopped
- 4 mackerel fillets (or use 2, if they are large)
- ½ tsp wholegrain mustard
- ½ tbsp clear honey
- ½ x 120g bag watercress, spinach and rocket salad
- 1 small shallot, thinly sliced

1 Finely crush the peppercorns and coriander seeds together using a pestle and mortar. Grate the zest from half an orange and mix into the pepper mixture with half the chopped chilli. Lightly slash the skin of the mackerel and press the zesty, peppery mixture on to the fish. Heat the grill to high.

2 For the oranges, slice the top and bottom off each, then cut away the peel and pith using a sharp knife. Holding each orange over a bowl to catch the juice, cut down either side of each segment to release it, then squeeze the pith for extra juice. Measure 2 tablespoon of juice into a small bowl and mix with the mustard, honey and remaining chilli.

3 Grill the mackerel, skin-side up, for 4 minutes or until crisp and cooked through. Meanwhile, divide the salad leaves between two plates and scatter with the orange segments and sliced shallot. Drizzle with the dressing and top with the grilled mackerel.

· ·
PER SERVING 412 kcals, protein 30g, carbs 18g, fat 25g, sat fat 5g, fibre 3g, sugar 17g, salt 0.32g

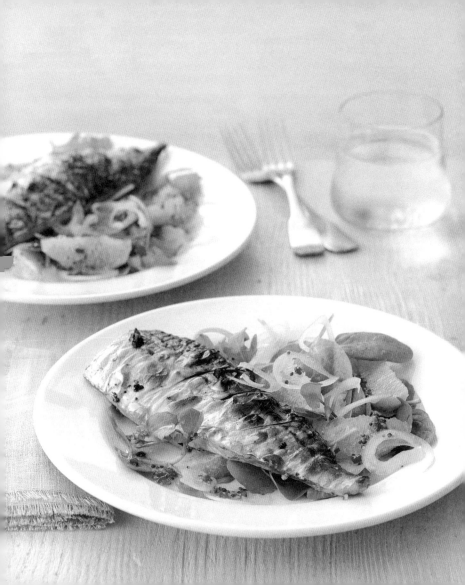

Fish parcels with romesco sauce & veg

Romesco is a Spanish sauce made from roasted peppers, almonds, chilli and garlic, often served with hake. Here we have paired it with less expensive cod fillets.

🕐 30 minutes 📋 2

- 2 firm white fish fillets (we used cod)
- 4 lemon slices
- 2 thyme sprigs
- 2 tbsp olive oil
- ½ cauliflower, cut into wedges
- 10 spring onions, ends trimmed, roots left intact
- 1 slice sourdough bread, torn into chunks
- 1 red chilli (deseeded, if you don't like it too hot)
- 2 garlic cloves, sliced
- 10 blanched almonds
- 2 ready-roasted red peppers, from a jar
- 1 tomato, peeled
- ½ tsp sherry vinegar

1 Heat oven to 200C/180C fan/gas 6. Put each fish fillet on a large piece of baking parchment and top each with a few slices of lemon and a sprig of thyme. Drizzle with 1 teaspoon of the oil and season. Fold over the top edges of each piece of parchment to make a seal, then scrunch up the ends like a sweet wrapper. Put the parcels on a baking sheet and bake in the oven for 15 minutes.

2 Meanwhile, steam the cauliflower for 4 minutes, then add the spring onions for 3 minutes more or until tender. Pat dry, then toss the veg in 2 teaspoons of the olive oil and season. In a large frying pan, toast the bread pieces in the remaining oil, then add the chilli and garlic, and cook for 1 minute. Tip into a food processor with the nuts, peppers, tomato and vinegar, and pulse until you have a rough paste. Season.

3 Wipe then heat the frying pan. Add the cauliflower wedges and spring onions, and cook for a few minutes for each side to brown. Serve alongside the fish and sauce.

PER SERVING 435 kcals, protein 38g, carbs 27g, fat 19g, sat fat 3g, fibre 6g, sugar 8g, salt 0.7g

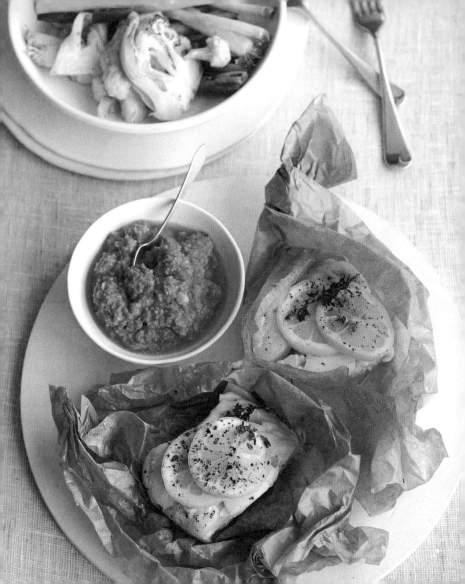

Piri-piri fish & chips with spicy peas

Give a traditional staple a spicy kick with some chilli marinade and minty peas. You can use any white fish. For an additional healthy side, serve with grilled tomatoes.

🕐 45 minutes 🥧 2

- 375g/13oz potatoes, cut into chips
- 1 tbsp olive oil
- juice ½ lemon
- 2 tbsp piri-piri marinade
- 300g/10oz frozen peas
- 1 green chilli, deseeded and finely chopped
- ½ garlic clove, crushed
- handful mint leaves, finely chopped
- 2 sea bass fillets

1 Heat oven to 200C/180C fan/gas 6. Toss the chips with half the olive oil and half the lemon juice, arrange in a layer in a roasting tin, then season. Cook for 25 minutes. Stir the remaining lemon juice into the marinade and set aside.

2 Meanwhile, bring a pan of water to the boil and cook the peas for 2–3 minutes, then drain. Return the peas to the empty pan and crush with the chilli, garlic, mint and the remaining oil. Season and keep warm.

3 After 25 minutes, turn the potatoes and move to the edges of the tin. Add the fish, skin-side up, and spoon over the marinade. Cook for another 10–12 minutes until the fish is cooked through. Serve with the crushed peas.

PER SERVING 450 kcals, protein 41g, carbs 47g, fat 11g, sat fat 2g, fibre 10g, sugar 6g, salt 1.2g

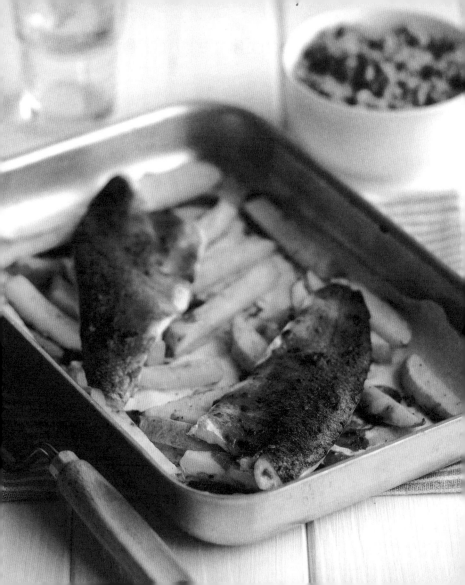

Sea bass en papillote with Thai flavours

. . . .

Make a parcel from baking parchment and let your fish steam to perfection while infusing with the fresh flavours of garlic, ginger, chilli and lime.

🕐 40 minutes   🥧 2

- 2 small sea bass, scaled and gutted
- 12 new potatoes, cleaned
- small knob salted butter
- coriander leaves, to garnish

FOR THE STUFFING
- 2 lemongrass stalks
- 3 garlic cloves
- 100g/4oz chunk ginger, finely sliced
- 3 small red chillies, finely chopped
- zest and juice 1 lime, plus extra wedges to garnish (optional)

1 Heat oven to 180C/160 fan/gas 4. First make the stuffing. Bruise the lemongrass by bashing it with the blunt side of a knife, then slice into thin rings. Squash the unpeeled garlic cloves to release their aroma and combine in a bowl with the remaining stuffing ingredients.

2 Place the fish on a 50cm/20in-long piece of baking parchment, laid across its width. Fill the stomach cavities with three-quarters of the stuffing, scattering the rest over the fish, then season. Fold the sides of the parchment over the heads and tails of the fish, then roll into a parcel. Put on a baking sheet and bake for 20–25 minutes, until the flesh flakes off the bone.

3 While the fish bakes, put the new potatoes in a pan of cold water and bring to the boil. Once cooked, drain well, slice in half and return to the pan with the butter.

4 Arrange the new potatoes and sea bass on two plates, in the parcels, if you like, and sprinkled with the coriander leaves and lime wedges to squeeze over, if you like.

. . . .
PER SERVING 361 kcals, protein 43g, carbs 29g, fat 8g, sat fat 2g, fibre 2g, sugar 4g, salt 0.7g

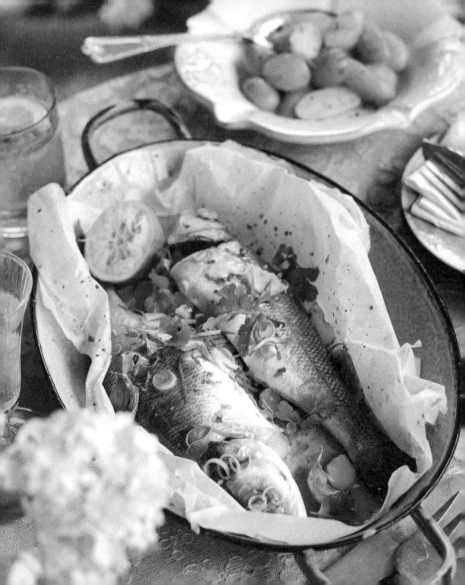

Tomato & tamarind fish curry

Use a sustainable white fish like hake and serve up this healthy Indian spice-pot with green beans and coriander that won't break your diet. It's great for entertaining.

🕐 35 minutes   🍽 4

- 6 garlic cloves
- 1 red chilli, roughly chopped (deseeded, if you don't like it too hot)
- thumb-sized piece ginger, peeled and roughly chopped
- 1 tsp ground turmeric
- 1 tbsp ground coriander
- 1 tbsp rapeseed oil
- 2 tsp cumin seeds
- 1 tsp fennel seeds
- 2 x 400g cans chopped tomatoes
- 200g/7oz green beans, trimmed and halved
- 1–2 tbsp tamarind paste
- 4 firm white skinless fish fillets (we used hake)
- handful coriander leaves, roughly chopped
- brown basmati rice, to serve

1. Blitz together the garlic, chilli, ginger, turmeric and ground coriander with 3 tablespoons water to make a paste. Heat the oil in a large pan with a lid and toast the cumin and fennel seeds, letting them sizzle until aromatic. Add the ginger paste and fry for 3 minutes.

2. Empty the tomatoes into the spice pan, plus a can of water. Add the beans, bring to the boil, then turn down the heat and simmer for 5 minutes. Stir in the tamarind paste. Add the fish fillets, generously season with ground black pepper, cover and simmer for 10 minutes. Take off the lid, carefully turn the fillets, then bubble the sauce until the fish is cooked through and the sauce is thick. Sprinkle over the coriander leaves and serve with rice.

PER SERVING 224 kcals, protein 31g, carbs 11g, fat 7g, sat fat 1g, fibre 4g, sugar 9g, salt 0.6g

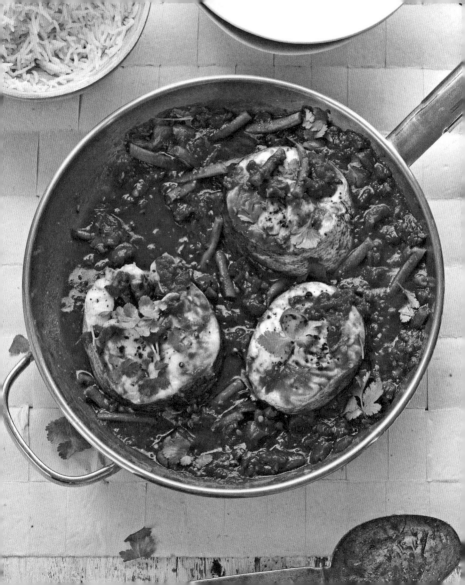

Asparagus & tuna salad

Give the bistro classic, Niçoise salad, a seasonal twist by swapping green beans for tender asparagus.

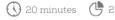 20 minutes 2

- 8 baby new potatoes
- 2 medium eggs
- 125g pack asparagus, woody ends removed
- 185g can tuna in spring water, drained and flaked into very large chunks
- small handful small black olives, halved
- 1 romaine lettuce, leaves torn into chunks

FOR THE DRESSING
- 1 shallot, finely chopped
- 1 tsp English mustard powder
- 2 tbsp white wine vinegar
- 1 tbsp extra-virgin olive oil
- pinch sugar

1 Boil the potatoes for 8–12 minutes until tender. Drain, cool a little under cold running water, then drain again well and set aside to finish cooling.

2 Put the eggs in a pan of cold water, bring to the boil and cook for 5 minutes. Then add the asparagus to the water and cook together for 2 minutes. Drain well and rinse everything under cold water to cool. Again drain asparagus well.

3 Once cool enough to handle, peel the eggs and halve or quarter. Whisk the dressing ingredients with 1 tablespoon water and some seasoning.

4 Tip the potatoes, asparagus, tuna, olives and lettuce into a bowl. Add the eggs, drizzle over the dressing, toss well to coat and serve.

PER SERVING 490 kcals, protein 36g, carbs 45g, fat 17g, sat fat 3g, fibre 10g, sugar 8g, salt 0.8g

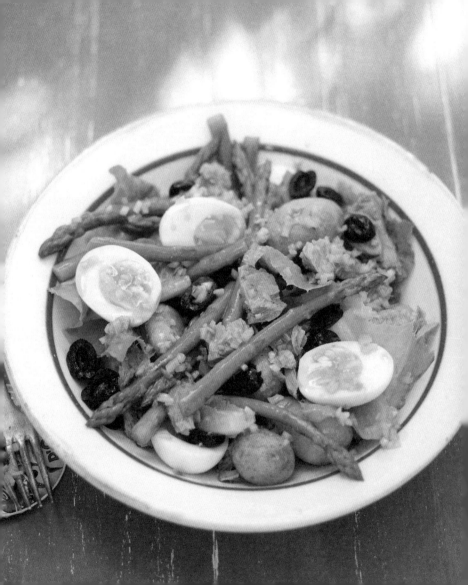

Citrus & ginger steamed fish with stir-fry veg

· · · · · · · · · · · · · · · · · · · ·

Try to eat white and oily fish at least once a week. Here, instead of being served with a carb like rice or pasta, this fish dish is accompanied by lightly cooked vegetables.

🕐 20 minutes   🍽 2

- zest and juice 1 orange
- 1 tbsp reduced-salt soy sauce
- 2 tsp white wine vinegar or rice vinegar
- 300g pack of 2 white fish fillets or loins (150g/5½oz each)
- 1 tbsp very finely shredded ginger
- 2 tsp sesame oil
- 10 spring onions halved and sliced lengthways
- 2 garlic cloves, thinly sliced
- 1 red pepper, deseeded and thinly sliced
- 150g/5½oz beansprouts
- 1–2 tsp toasted sesame seeds

1 Mix the orange juice and zest with the soy and vinegar in a small bowl to make a dressing. Line the top of a steamer with baking paper and heat water in the base. Top the fish fillets with a little of the ginger then arrange them in the steamer, spoon 2 tablespoons of the dressing over the fish then cover and steam of 5–6 minutes until the fish flakes easily when tested.

2 Meanwhile, heat the sesame oil in a non-stick wok then stir-fry the onions, garlic, pepper and remaining ginger for 2 minutes. Add the beansprouts and cook for 2 minutes more. Pour any juices from the fish into the vegetables. Stir through the remaining dressing then divide the veg between bowls, top with the fish and scatter with the seeds.

· ·

PER SERVING 259 kcals, protein 33g, carbs 14g, fat 7g, sat fat 1g, fibre 5g, sugar 11g, salt 1.2g

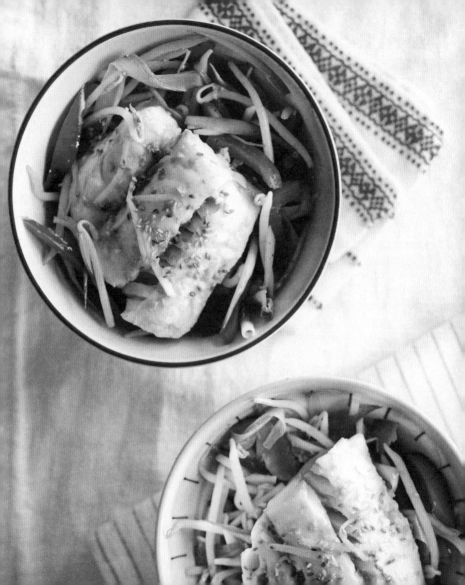

Corn & green-bean cakes with avocado & chilli jam

. . . .

Vegetarian fritters made with sweetcorn, spring onions and green beans, served with chilli-and-coriander avocado salsa and a sweet dipping sauce. Delicious.

 20 minutes 2

- 200g/7oz sweetcorn kernels, boiled, then drained (or use a 198g can)
- 2 spring onions, chopped
- 25g/1oz green beans, chopped into 1cm/½in pieces
- ½–1 red chilli (deseeded, if you don't like it too hot), finely chopped
- handful coriander leaves
- 50g/2oz self-raising flour
- 1 egg, beaten
- 40ml/1½fl oz milk
- 1 small avocado, diced
- juice ½ lime
- 1 tbsp rapeseed oil
- ½ x 250g jar chilli jam

1 Put the sweetcorn, spring onions, beans, half of the chilli and coriander, the flour, eggs, milk and some seasoning in a large bowl. Mix together, then set aside. Mix the avocado with the remaining chilli and coriander, the lime juice and some seasoning to make a salsa.

2 Heat the oil in a large non-stick frying pan. Spoon in mounds of the corn mixture, slightly spaced apart. When browned on the underside, turn over and cook for a further 1–2 minutes. Serve the corn-and-bean cakes with the avocado salsa and the chilli jam.

. . . .
PER SERVING 353 kcals, protein 9g, carbs 35g, fat 20g, sat fat 4g, fibre 5g, sugar 8g, salt 0.8g

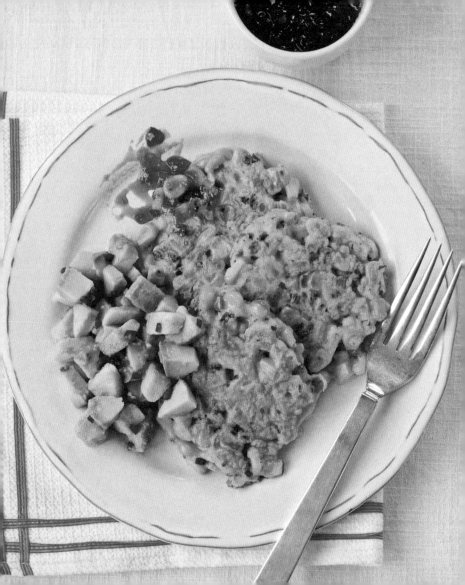

Orzo with spinach & cherry tomatoes

A tiny rice-shaped variety of pasta makes this dish almost like risotto. It's quick, healthy, filling and suitable for vegetarians.

🕐 30 minutes 📂 2

- 200g/7oz orzo
- 1 tbsp olive or rapeseed oil
- ½ celery heart, chopped
- 1 small red onion, chopped
- 2 garlic cloves, chopped
- 400g can cherry tomatoes
- 125g/4½oz baby leaf spinach
- 10 pitted black olives, halved
- small handful dill, leaves chopped
- small handful mint, leaves chopped

1 Cook the orzo according to the pack instructions. Drain, rinse under cold water, drain again and toss with half the oil. Set aside.

2 Meanwhile, heat the remaining oil in a large sauté pan. Add the celery, onion and some seasoning, and cook for 8 minutes until soft. Add the garlic, cook for 1 minute, then tip in the cherry tomatoes and simmer for 10 minutes.

3 Add the spinach to the pan, cover with a lid to wilt the leaves, then add the orzo, olives, dill and mint. Season and serve straight away

PER SERVING 471 kcals, protein 16g, carbs 81g, fat 9g, sat fat 1g, fibre 5g, sugar 10g, salt 1.2g

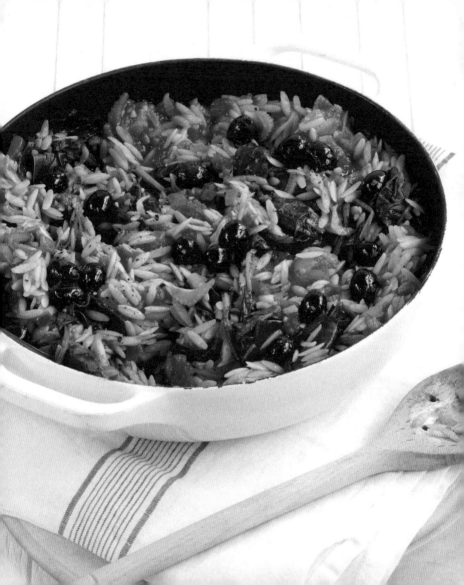

Baked potatoes with spicy dhal

· · · · · · · · · · · · · · · · · · · ·

Cook red lentils with cumin, mustard seeds and turmeric, and serve in a fluffy jacket potato with chutney. Curcumin in turmeric is thought to fight age-related decline.

🕐 1 hour 10 minutes   🥧 2

- 2 baking potatoes (Vivaldi have a lovely creamy texture)
- 1 tbsp rapeseed oil
- ½ tsp each cumin seeds, black mustard seeds and ground turmeric
- 1 onion, thinly sliced
- 3 garlic cloves, sliced
- 1 red chilli, deseeded and sliced
- 85g/3oz red split lentils
- 1 tomato, chopped
- 400ml/14fl oz vegetable stock
- 210g can chickpeas, drained and rinsed
- good handful chopped coriander leaves
- mango chutney or lime pickle, to serve

1 Heat oven to 200C/180C fan/gas 6. Put the potatoes in the oven and bake for 1 hour until tender and the skin is crispy.

2 While the potatoes are baking, make the dhal. Heat the oil in a medium pan and fry the spices to release their flavours. As soon as they start to crackle, tip in the onion, garlic and chilli, with a splash of water to stop the spices from burning. Cook for 5 minutes until the onion softens.

3 Add the lentils, tomato and stock, then cover and cook for 10 minutes. Tip in the chickpeas, cover and cook for 10 minutes more until the lentils are tender. Season the dhal to taste, stir in the coriander and spoon on to the jacket potatoes. Serve with mango chutney or lime pickle.

· ·
PER SERVING 556 kcals, protein 23g, carbs 96g, fat 8g, sat fat 1g, fibre 12g, sugar 10g, salt 1.1g

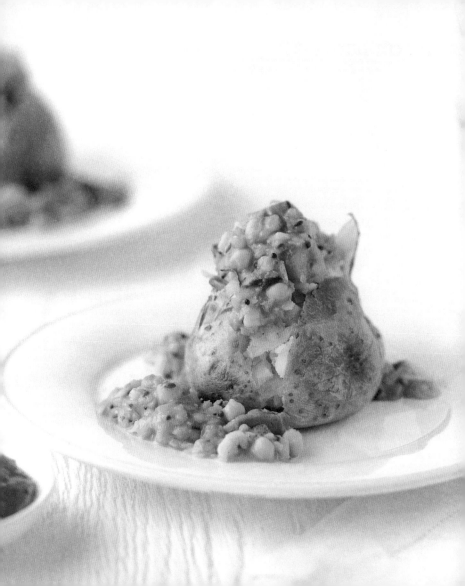

Bhaji frittata

· ·

Perfect for a lunchbox or picnic, or with a salad for supper, this dish takes a Mediterranean-style omelette and adds some Indian flavours, potatoes and peas.

🕐 40 minutes   🍽 4

- 2 tbsp rapeseed oil
- 2 onions, thinly sliced
- 1 garlic clove, finely chopped
- 2 tsp mild curry powder
- 450g/1lb potatoes, coarsely grated and any excess liquid squeezed out
- 6 medium eggs, beaten
- 100g/4oz frozen peas
- small pack coriander, leaves roughly chopped
- mango chutney, low-fat natural bio yogurt and naan bread, to serve (optional)

1 Heat oven to 200C/180C fan/gas 6. Heat the oil in an ovenproof frying pan and fry the onion for about 10 minutes over a medium heat until golden. Add the garlic and curry powder, and cook for 1–2 minutes.

2 Next, add the grated potatoes and cook for 5–8 minutes, stirring occasionally. You want the potatoes not only to soften but also catch a little and turn golden in patches. Season the eggs, then pour into the pan with the peas and most of the coriander, swirling to coat the potato mixture. Cook for 1 minute more, then transfer to the oven for 10 minutes until the eggs have set.

3 Sprinkle with the remaining coriander and serve with mango chutney, natural yogurt and naan bread, if you like.

· ·

PER SERVING 282 kcals, protein 13g, carbs 27g, fat 14g, sat fat 3g, fibre 6g, sugar 5g, salt 0.3g

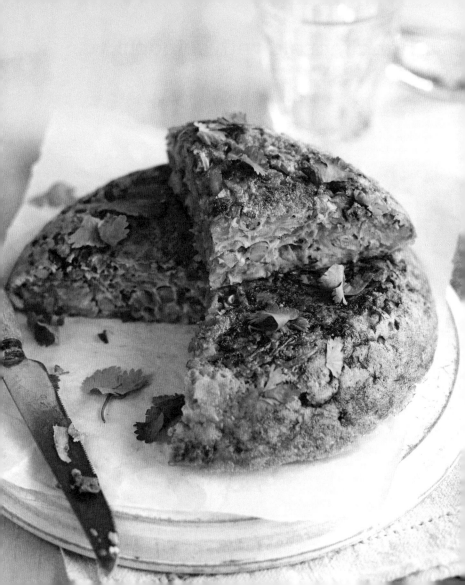

Chana masala with spinach

A superhealthy vegetable-packed curry with chickpeas, spinach and tomatoes. Serve with filling brown basmati rice.

 35 minutes 2

- 75g/2½oz quick-cook brown basmati rice
- 1 tsp cumin seeds
- 1 tbsp rapeseed oil
- 1 medium onion, finely chopped
- 1 garlic clove, finely chopped
- 1cm/½in piece ginger, peeled and finely chopped or grated
- ½ red chilli, deseeded and finely chopped
- 1 tsp ground coriander
- 1 tsp ground cumin
- 1 tsp ground turmeric
- 1 tsp paprika
- 1 tsp garam masala
- 400g can whole plum tomatoes
- 400g can chickpeas, drained and rinsed
- juice ½ lemon
- 220g bag baby leaf spinach

1 Cook the rice according to the pack instructions. Meanwhile, heat a large non-stick pan or wok and dry-fry the cumin seeds for 1 minute, stirring often, while they pop. Remove to a bowl.

2 Using the same pan or wok, heat the oil, add the onion, garlic, ginger and chilli, and sauté over a medium heat for about 3 minutes. Reduce the heat, add all the spices, stir well and cook for a further 2 minutes. Add the tomatoes, stirring, and use the side of a spoon to break them up into smaller bite-sized chunks. Add the chickpeas and 200ml/7fl oz water.

3 Bring to the boil, then simmer for 10 minutes before stirring in the lemon juice and spinach. Let the spinach wilt, then remove the pan or wok from the heat.

4 Divide the rice between two bowls and serve the curry. (The flavours intensify as it cools, so for a fuller flavour, make earlier in the day and reheat slowly prior to serving.)

PER SERVING 420 kcals, protein 20g, carbs 60g, fat 12g, sat fat 1g, fibre 12g, sugar 12g, salt 1.3g

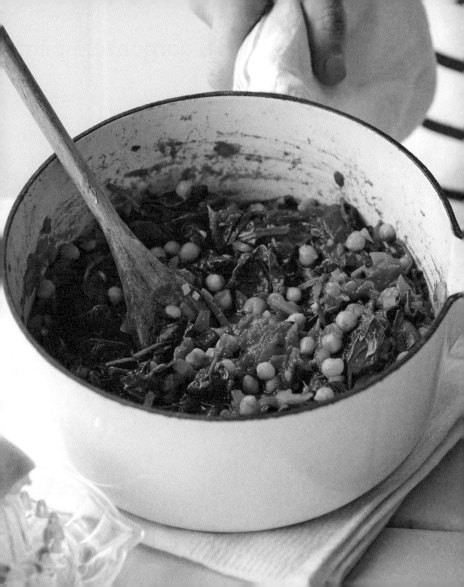

Squash, mushroom & gorgonzola pilaf

Deliciously savoury and filling, and surprisingly low in calories as a little strong-flavoured cheese goes a long way.

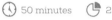 50 minutes 2

- 1 tsp rapeseed oil
- 1 large onion, halved and sliced
- 3 garlic cloves, finely chopped
- 200g/7oz chunk butternut squash, peeled, deseeded and diced
- 140g/5oz button mushrooms
- 125g/4½oz brown basmati rice
- 700ml/1¼ pints reduced-salt vegetable stock
- 10 pieces dried mushrooms, chopped
- 2 tsp chopped sage leaves
- small pack parsley leaves and stalks separated, chopped
- 40g/1½oz gorgonzola, crumbled

1 Heat the oil in a large non-stick pan, add the onion and garlic, and fry for 5 minutes. Tip in the squash and mushrooms, and cook a few minutes more. Stir in the rice, then pour in the stock. Stir well, then add the dried mushrooms, sage and parsley stalks. Cover and simmer over a low heat for 35–40 minutes until the rice is tender. Check towards the end of cooking and add a little water if the rice has absorbed all the stock.

2 Remove from the heat, fold in the parsley leaves and the cheese with a grinding of black pepper then allow to stand for 5 minutes before serving.

PER SERVING 422 kcals, protein 17g, carbs 63g, fat 10g, sat fat 5g, fibre 10g, sugar 13g, salt 0.9g

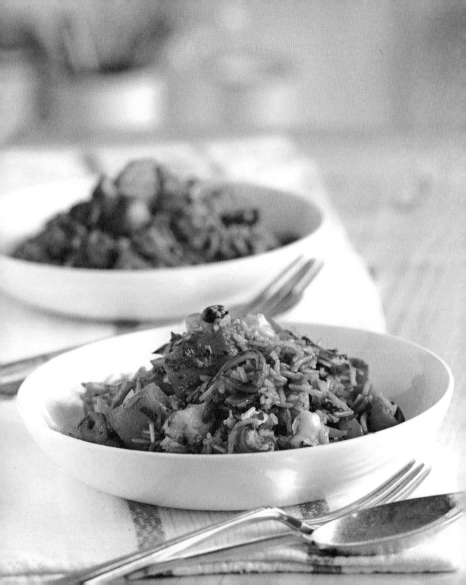

Veggie Bolognese with Quorn

Quorn is a low-fat veggie alternative to meat, which is made from a fungi related to mushrooms. It works really well in this filling Bolognese sauce that will feed the family

🕐 40 minutes   🅿 4

- 1–2 tbsp rapeseed or olive oil
- 1 carrot, diced
- 1 onion, halved and finely chopped
- 200g pack mushrooms, sliced
- 2 garlic cloves, chopped
- 400g can chopped tomatoes
- 1 tsp dried mixed herbs
- 1 tbsp tomato purée or 2 tbsp tomato ketchup
- 1 tbsp vegetable stock powder
- 350g pack Quorn mince
- 350g/12oz spaghetti, preferably wholewheat
- vegetarian Parmesan, to garnish
- salad, to serve

1 Heat the oil in a large frying pan, add the carrot and onion, and cook over a medium heat, stirring frequently, for about 10 minutes until the onion is soft. Add the mushrooms and garlic, and stir-fry for a few minutes more.

2 Tip the tomatoes into the pan with half a can of water, the herbs, tomato purée or ketchup and stock powder, then stir well to make a sauce. Stir the Quorn into the sauce, season, then cover and simmer for 12 minutes until the vegetables are cooked and the mixture is saucy rather than wet.

3 Meanwhile, bring a large pan of salted water to the boil. Add the spaghetti and boil according to the pack instructions – usually about 9–10 minutes – until just tender. Drain the spaghetti and pile into four bowls. Spoon the sauce on top, then generously grate over the cheese. Serve with a salad.

PER SERVING 465 kcals, protein 28g, carbs 63g, fat 9g, sat fat 1g, fibre 11g, sugar 10g, salt 1.3g

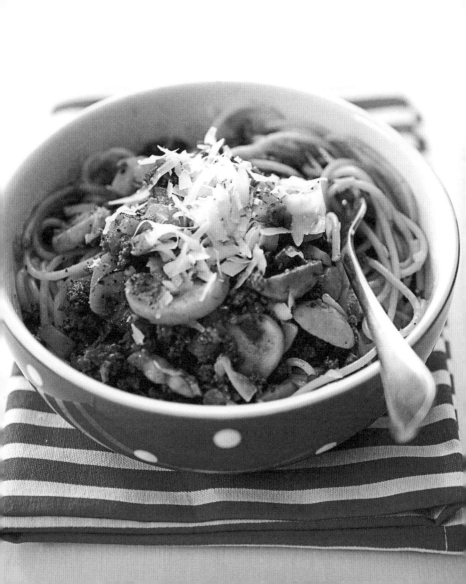

Aubergine tagine with lemon & mint & almond couscous

Almonds in the couscous add extra protein to this veggie supper. Freeze what you don't eat and halve the couscous mixture, if serving two.

🕐 30 minutes 📤 4

- 1 tbsp rapeseed oil
- 1 large onion, chopped
- 3 garlic cloves, chopped
- 1 tbsp harissa paste
- 1 tsp cumin seeds
- ½ tsp ground cinnamon
- 200ml/7fl oz reduced-salt vegetable stock
- 400g can chopped tomatoes
- 350g/12oz baby aubergines, trimmed and slit a few times
- 2 strips lemon zest, finely chopped
- 390g can butter beans, drained and rinsed
- 175g/6oz wholemeal couscous
- 40g/1½oz toasted flaked almonds
- 150g pot 0%-fat probiotic natural yogurt
- mint leaves, to garnish

1 Heat the oil in a large non-stick pan and fry the onion and garlic for 5 minutes. Stir in the harissa, cumin and cinnamon, cook briefly then tip in the stock and tomatoes.

2 Add the aubergines and lemon then cover the pan and cook gently for 15–20 minutes until the aubergines are meltingly tender. Add the butter beans to the tagine and warm through.

3 Meanwhile, cook the couscous according to the pack instructions, then stir in the almonds Serve with a spoonful of yogurt on top and garnish with a few mint leaves.

PER SERVING 361 kcals, protein 16g, carbs 50g, fat 10g, sat fat 1g, fibre 9g, sugar 12g, salt 0.9g

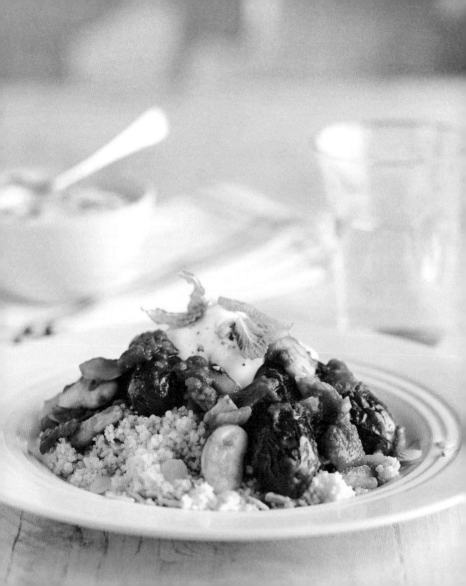

Smoky sweet-potato bean cakes with citrus salad

· ·

These spicy chipotle cakes are not only thrifty but they also count as four of your 5-a-day of fruit and vegetables.

 30–35 minutes   2

- 1 sweet potato (about 200g/7oz), cut into cubes
- 400g can red kidney beans, drained and rinsed
- 3 spring onions, finely sliced
- small bunch coriander, leaves chopped
- 1 tbsp chipotle paste
- 2 tbsp rapeseed oil
- 2 tbsp low-fat mayonnaise
- juice 1 lime
- 1 Little Gem lettuce, torn
- ½ cucumber, halved lengthways and sliced on the diagonal
- 1 carrot, halved lengthways and sliced on the diagonal

1 Microwave the sweet potato on High for 6 minutes until tender. Lightly mash the bean then add the potato, 2 of the sliced spring onions, the coriander, chipotle paste and some seasoning. Mash a little more until the potato is combined. Shape into four cakes.

2 Heat the oil in a non-stick frying pan, then fry the bean cakes for 4–5 minutes each side.

3 Meanwhile, mix the mayo, lime juice and some seasoning in a bowl. Add the remaining spring onion and the salad ingredients, and toss well. Serve the citrus salad alongside the bean cakes, and drizzle the bean cakes with a little of the mayo, if you like.

· ·

PER SERVING 431 kcals, protein 24g, carbs 39g, fat 24g, sat fat 3g, fibre 10g, sugar 15g, salt 1.4g

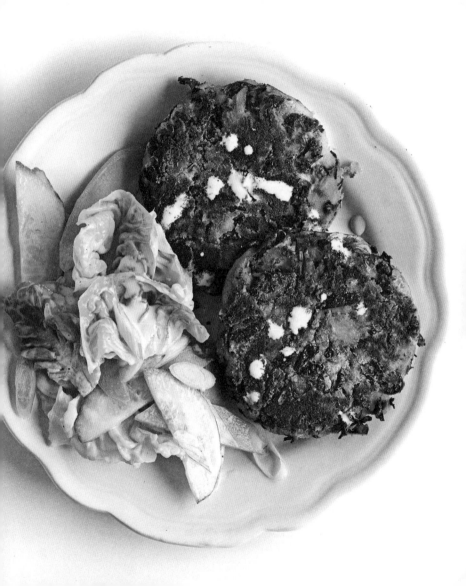

Puy lentils with smoked tofu

Benefit from the slow-release energy of lentils combined with the rich flavour of smoked tofu, paprika and sweet peppers.

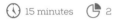 15 minutes   2

- 1-cal oil spray, for frying
- 1 large courgette, finely diced
- 100g/4oz smoked tofu, finely diced
- ½ tsp smoked paprika
- 1½ tbsp balsamic vinegar
- 250g sachet cooked Puy lentils
- 1 red onion, finely chopped
- 1 medium roasted red pepper from a jar (not in oil), about 85g/3oz, sliced
- good handful pea shoots or rocket leaves

1 Spray a non-stick pan with three sprays of the oil and add the courgette, tofu and smoked paprika. Cook for a few minutes to soften the courgettes. Stir in the balsamic vinegar and allow to sizzle and reduce.

2 Meanwhile, tip the lentils, onion and pepper into a bowl and toss gently to break up any clumps of lentils. Add the tofu and courgettes, and toss again. Scatter over the pea shoots or rocket leaves just before serving.

PER SERVING 300 kcals, protein 24g, carbs 38g, fat 6g, sat fat 1g, fibre 12g, sugar 8g, salt 1.3g

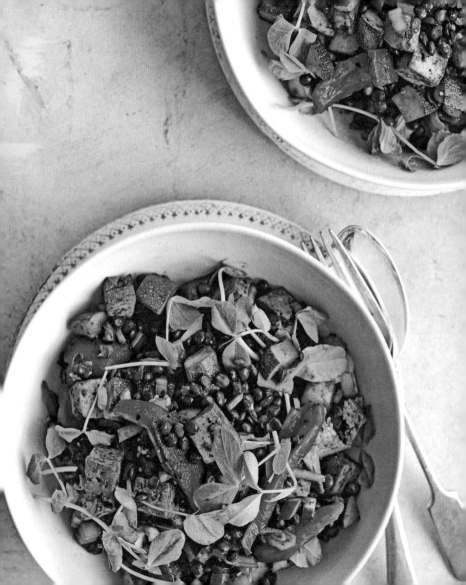

Spicy bean tostadas with pickled onions & radish salad

Tex-Mex goes healthy with these corn tortillas topped with chipotle kidney beans, pickled red onions, coriander and lime.

🕐 27 minutes 　 🍴 2

- 2 red onions, 1 thinly sliced, 1 finely chopped
- 2 limes, juice 1 and 1 cut into wedges
- 1½ tbsp rapeseed oil
- 2 garlic cloves, finely chopped
- 2 tsp ground cumin
- 1 tbsp tomato purée
- 1 tbsp chipotle paste
- 400g can kidney beans, drained and rinsed
- 4 corn tortillas
- 140g/5oz radishes, thinly sliced
- large handful coriander, roughly chopped

1 Heat oven to 220C/200C fan/gas 7. Put the sliced onion, lime juice and seasoning in a bowl, and set aside.

2 Heat 1 tablespoon of the oil in a pan and fry the chopped onion and garlic until tender. Stir in the cumin and fry for 1 minute more. Add the tomato purée, chipotle paste and beans, stir, then tip in half a can of water. Simmer for 5 minutes, season, then roughly mash to a purée. (You can cook for a few minutes more if it is a bit runny, or add a few splashes of water to thin.)

3 Meanwhile, brush the tortillas with the remaining oil and place on a baking sheet. Bake for 8 minutes until crisp. Spread the tortillas with the bean mixture. Mix the radishes and coriander with the pickled onions, then spoon on top. Serve with lime wedges.

PER SERVING 488 kcals, protein 16g, carbs 68g, fat 10g, sat fat 4g, fibre 12g, sugar 14g, salt 1.4g

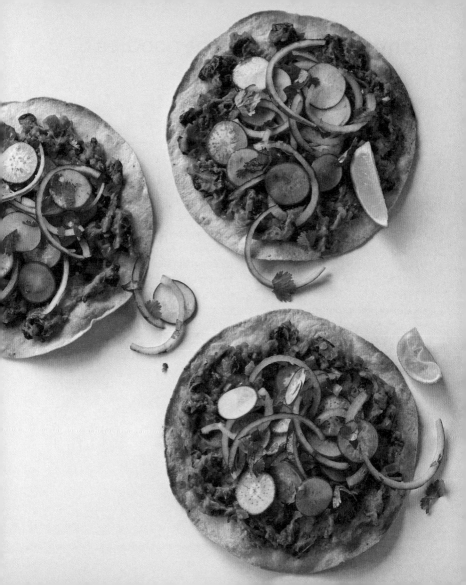

Lamb with buckwheat noodles & tomato dressing

Take care adding the fish sauce as it is high in salt. Red meat has a bad reputation, but provided it is lean, not too large a portion and not eaten every day, it is fine.

 20 minutes   2

- 12 cherry tomatoes, quartered
- 1 tsp Thai fish sauce
- zest and juice 1 lime
- 1 tbsp sweet chilli sauce
- 100g/4oz buckwheat noodles
- 2 tsp rapeseed oil
- 1 red onion, halved and sliced
- 1 carrot, cut into matchsticks
- 1 red pepper, deseeded and sliced
- 100g/4oz shredded white cabbage
- 200g/7oz lean lamb loin fillet or steaks, diced
- 4 tbsp chopped mint leaves

1 Lightly squash the tomatoes with the fish sauce, lime juice and zest and the chilli sauce to make the dressing. Cook the noodles according to the pack instructions.

2 Meanwhile, heat the oil in a wok and stir-fry the onion, carrot and pepper for 5 minutes or until softening. Add the cabbage and cook for a few minutes more. Push the veg to one side of the wok then add the lamb and cook briefly so that it is cooked but still tender and juicy. Take the wok from the heat, toss in the noodles, tomato dressing and mint, and serve.

PER SERVING 477 kcals, protein 30g, carbs 60g, fat 12g, sat fat 3g, fibre 8g, sugar 22g, salt 1.2g

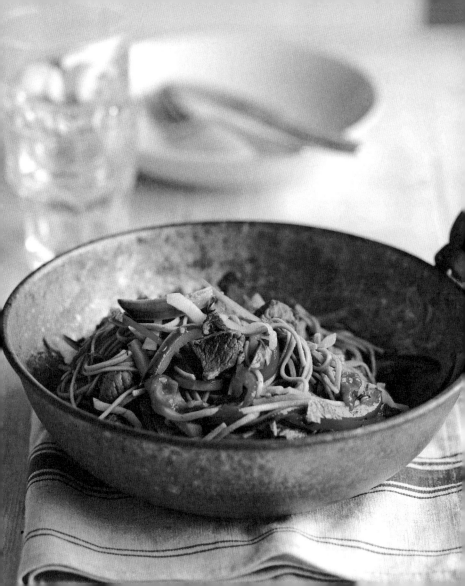

Steak, roasted-pepper & pearl-barley salad

· · · · · · · · · · · · · · · · · · · ·

A vibrant salad packed with yellow and red peppers, colourful onion, beef cooked to your liking and healthy grains.

🕐 40 minutes   🍽 2

- 85g/3oz pearl barley, rinsed
- 1 red pepper, deseeded and cut into strips
- 1 yellow pepper, deseeded and cut into strips
- 1 red onion, cut into 8 wedges, leaving root intact
- 1 tbsp olive oil, plus a little extra
- 1 large lean beef steak, about 300g/10oz, trimmed of any excess fat
- ½ x 100g bag watercress, roughly chopped
- juice ½ lemon, plus wedges to garnish (optional)

1 Put the pearl barley in a large pan of water. Bring to the boil and cook vigorously for 25–30 minutes or until tender. Drain thoroughly and transfer to a bowl. Set aside.

2 Meanwhile, heat oven to 200C/180C fan/gas 6. Put the peppers in a roasting tin with the onion wedges, toss in the olive oil and roast for about 20 minutes until tender.

3 While the peppers are roasting, rub the steak with a little bit of extra oil and season. Cook in a non-stick frying pan for 3–4 minutes each side, or to your liking. Leave to rest for a few minutes.

4 Mix the cooked peppers and onions into the barley. Stir though the watercress, lemon juice and some seasoning, then transfer to a serving plate. Thinly slice the steaks, put on top of the salad and serve with lemon wedges to squeeze over, if you like.

· ·

PER SERVING 498 kcals, protein 38g, carbs 48g, fat 17g, sat fat 5g, fibre 6g, sugar 13g, salt 0.2g

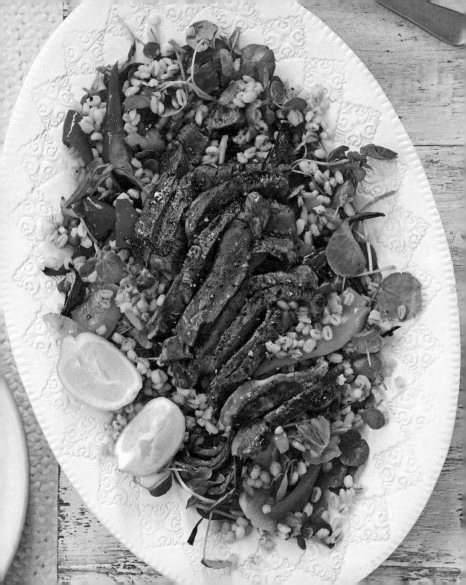

Seared steak with celery & pepper caponata

Lean red meat is rich in iron, B vitamins and zinc, as well as protein, so this recipe is a healthy option when eaten in moderation.

 40 minutes   2

- 200g/7oz extra-lean beef fillet steak
- 140g/5oz spinach

FOR THE CAPONATA
- 1-cal oil spray, for frying
- 1 red onion, halved and sliced
- 2 garlic cloves, cut into slivers
- 400g can chopped tomatoes
- 2 celery sticks, sliced
- 1 orange pepper, deseeded, quartered and sliced
- 25g/1oz pitted Kalamata olives, halved (about 8)
- 1 tbsp capers
- ½ tsp dried oregano or 1 tbsp fresh
- 1 tsp balsamic vinegar

1 Spray a large, wide non-stick pan with three sprays of the oil then add the onions and garlic for the caponata, cover and cook for 5 minutes, stirring halfway through to brown them.

2 Tip in the tomatoes and a can of water, then stir in all the other caponata ingredients. Cover the pan and leave to simmer for 30 minutes.

3 Heat a griddle or small non-stick frying pan to high. Generously grind black pepper over the steak then sear it on both sides until cooked to your liking – about 6 minutes. Allow to rest while you wilt the spinach in a covered pan.

4 Spoon the caponata into the centre of serving plates, top with the spinach then slice the beef and arrange on top to serve.

PER SERVING 269 kcals, protein 27g, carbs 19g, fat 10g, sat fat 3, fibre 9g, sugar 15g, salt 1.1g

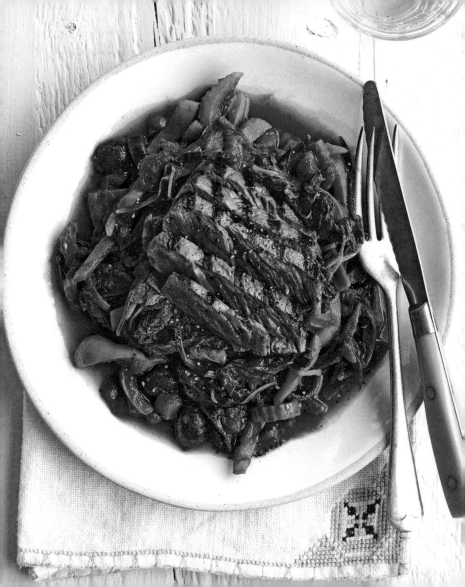

Thai burgers with sweet-potato chips & pineapple salsa

Sweet-potato chips make a great side to these tasty burgers and make up part of your 5-a-day, unlike potatoes. Pineapple canned in juice is fine if you don't have fresh.

🕐 50 minutes   🥧 2

- 2 sweet potatoes, unpeeled and cut into chunky chips
- ½ tbsp rapeseed or olive oil
- 500g/1lb 2oz extra-lean minced pork or beef
- 1 tbsp Thai red curry paste
- 3 spring onions, chopped
- ½ small bunch coriander, leaves chopped
- 100g/4oz pineapple chunks, diced
- generous squeeze lime
- 1 red chilli, deseeded and finely chopped
- 1 tbsp sweet chilli sauce, plus extra for dipping chips
- 2 buns, toasted
- ½ Little Gem lettuce

1 Heat oven to 200C/180C fan/gas 6. Toss the sweet-potato chips with the oil and some seasoning on a baking sheet. Roast for 40–45 minutes until golden and crisp.

2 Mix the mince with the curry paste, half the spring onions, half the coriander and some seasoning. Shape into four burgers. Set aside.

3 Mix the remaining spring onions and coriander with the pineapple, lime juice, red chilli and sweet chilli sauce to make a salsa.

4 When the chips have 10 minutes to go, heat a non-stick frying pan or griddle to high and cook the burgers for 3–5 minutes on each side until golden and cooked through. Serve the burgers in the buns with lettuce leaves and the salsa piled on top; the sweet-potato chips and some extra chilli sauce for dipping.

PER SERVING 491 kcals, protein 26g, carbs 61g, fat 15g, sat fat 4g, fibre 7g, sugar 19g, salt 1.5g

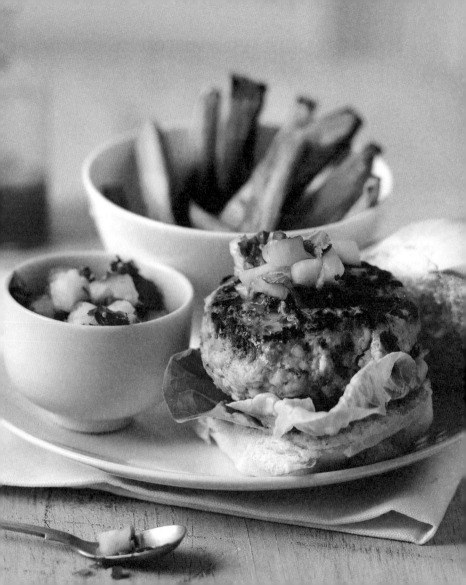

Herb roast pork with vegetable roasties & apple gravy

Entertaining this weekend? Try this healthy roast with Savoy cabbage and peas.

 2 hours 5 minutes   6

- 1.25kg/2lb 12oz boneless pork leg roasting joint
- 1 tbsp grainy mustard
- 2 tbsp each chopped parsley and thyme, plus extra sprigs
- 1 tsp chopped sage leaves
- 80g pack Parma ham
- 1-cal oil spray, for roasting
- 3 carrots, halved lengthways then cut across
- 6 small potatoes (about 500g/1lb 2oz), halved
- 2 red onions, cut into wedges
- 12 garlic cloves
- 1 small celeriac (650g/1lb 6oz), peeled and cut into 12 wedges
- 2 tbsp cornflour
- 600ml/1 pint reduced-salt chicken stock
- 1 small Bramley apple, diced

1 Heat oven to 180C/160C fan/gas 4. Cut and discard all the rind and fat from the pork. Spread the pork with the mustard, scatter with the chopped herbs and season with black pepper. Put the ham slices on top of the pork to protect the meat.

2 Spray a large roasting tin with the oil and put the pork in the centre. Surround with the vegetables and thyme sprigs, then spray and cover with foil. Roast for 1 hour, then uncover, spray again and roast for 20 minutes more.

3 Meanwhile, mix the cornflour with a little water to make a paste, heat the stock in a pan, stir in the cornflour and cook, stirring, until thickened. Add the apple and cook for 5 minutes until softened but holds its shape.

4 Remove the meat from the tin, pour any juices into the apple gravy then raise the oven to 220C/200C fan/gas 7. Spray the veg with oil and roast for 20 minutes more, as the meat rests, to brown them. Serve the pork with the roast and fresh veg and apple gravy.

PER SERVING 418 kcals, protein 50g, carbs 30g, fat 11g, sat fat 3g, fibre 7g, sugar 10g, salt 1.4g

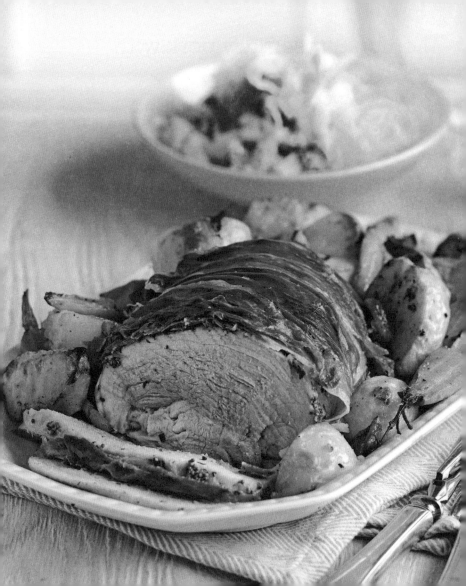

Lemon & rosemary pork with chickpea salad

. . . .

Chickpeas make a great accompaniment and are also fast to prepare, so this satisfying dish is on the table in 20 minutes, if you don't marinate the pork.

 20 minutes   2

- ½ tbsp rapeseed or olive oil
- 1 tsp chopped rosemary leaves
- 2 garlic cloves, crushed
- juice and zest ½ small lemon
- 2 boneless pork steaks, trimmed of excess fat
- 1 small red onion, finely sliced
- 1 tbsp sherry vinegar
- 400g chickpeas, drained and rinsed
- 2 large handfuls mixed salad leaves including rocket

1 Mix the oil, rosemary, garlic, lemon juice and zest in a large bowl. Add the pork, turn to coat and season. If you have time, marinate in the fridge for 30 minutes.

2 Heat a large non-stick frying pan. Lift the pork out of the marinade, shaking off any excess and reserving the marinade for later. Cook the pork in the pan for 3–4 minutes each side or until cooked through. Rest the pork on a plate while you make the salad.

3 Pour the reserved marinade into the pan with the onion. Cook for 1 minute over a high heat before adding the vinegar, plus 2 tablespoons water. Bubble down for 1 minute, until the onion has softened a little and the dressing has thickened slightly. Stir through the chickpeas and any of the resting juices from the pork.

4 Put the salad leaves into a bowl, tip in the pan contents and gently toss, before eating immediately with the pork.

. . . .

PER SERVING 396 kcals, protein 40g, carbs 23g, fat 17g, sat fat 3g, fibre 6g, sugar 3g, salt 0.9g

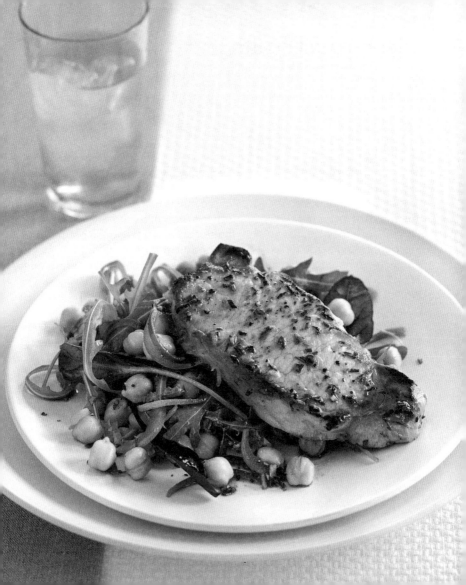

Spiced roast fruits

· · · · · · · · · · · · · · · · · · · ·

Perfect for entertaining, figs and peaches roast beautifully with honey and spices.

 55 minutes   6

- 4 bay leaves
- 2 cinnamon sticks
- 1 vanilla pod
- 4 seeds from ½ star anise
- zest and juice 3 oranges
- 4 tbsp clear honey
- 3 tbsp light muscovado sugar
- 6 peaches or nectarines
- 6 figs
- 25g/1oz unsalted butter
- crème fraîche or low-fat Greek yogurt and macaroons or soft Amaretti biscuits, to serve (optional)

1 The day before: tear the bay leaves and break the cinnamon into two or three pieces to release the oils and perfumes. Split the vanilla pod in half and scrape out the seeds with the back of a knife. Mix in a bowl with the star anise seeds and the pepper, orange zest and juice, honey and sugar to make a sauce. Cover and chill until ready to serve.

2 Half an hour before serving, heat oven to 200C/180C fan/gas 6. Cut the peaches or nectarines in half and remove the stones. Halve the figs. Put the peaches or nectarines skin-side down in a large baking dish or a roasting tin with sides. Pour the spicy sauce over the fruit and dot with the butter. Roast in the oven for 10 minutes, add the figs and baste the fruits with a large spoon. Roast for 15 minutes more, basting at least three times, until the fruits are tender.

3 Serve the fruits with crème fraîche or Greek yogurt and macaroons or Amaretti biscuits to soak up all the lovely juices.

· · · · · · · · · · · · · · · · · · · ·
PER SERVING 160 kcals, protein 2g, carbs 32g, fat 4g, sat fat 2g, fibre 3g, sugar 15g, salt none

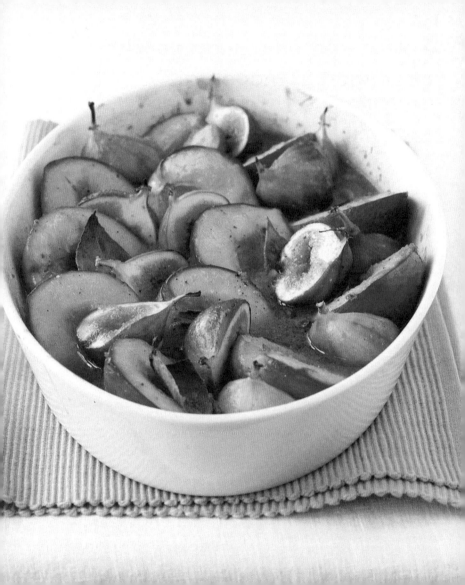

Spiced-glazed pineapple with cinnamon fromage frais

Try this tropical treat when you want to end a meal on a sweet note without too much effort or too many calories.

🕐 20 minutes 🍴 4

- zest and juice 1 lime
- 2 tbsp clear honey
- 2 pinches ground cinnamon
- few gratings nutmeg
- 2 tsp icing sugar, sifted
- 200g/7oz very low-fat fromage frais
- 2 tsp butter
- 1 pineapple, cut into 8 long wedges, skin and core removed

1 Mix the lime juice and half the zest in a bowl with 1 tablespoon of the honey and a pinch each of cinnamon and nutmeg to make a spiced lime sauce. In another small bowl, stir the icing sugar into the fromage frais and dust with the remaining pinch of cinnamon.

2 Heat the butter and remaining honey in a non-stick frying pan until melted. Add the pineapple and cook over a high heat for 8 minutes, turning regularly until caramelised Pour in the spiced lime sauce and bubble for a few seconds, tossing the pineapple to glaze in the sauce.

3 Serve the spiced-glazed pineapple immediately, sprinkled with the remaining lime zest and accompanied by a dollop of the cinnamon fromage frais.

PER SERVING 159 kcals, protein 5g, carbs 31g, fat 3g, sat fat 1g, fibre 2g, sugar 30g, salt 0.1g

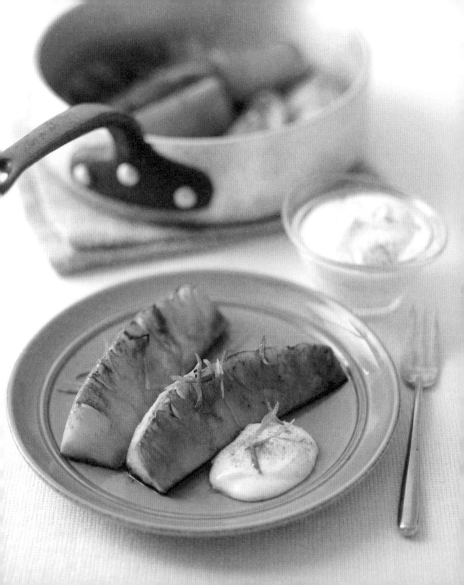

Oeufs au lait

. . . .

These little French vanilla-custard puddings are deliciously creamy and surprisingly low in fat.

🕐 40 minutes, plus chilling 🥧 4

- butter, for greasing
- 425ml/14fl oz milk
- 85g/3oz caster sugar
- 1 sachet vanilla sugar or 1 tsp vanilla extract
- 2 eggs

1 Butter four ramekins, about 150ml each. Heat oven to 160C/140C fan/gas 3. Have a roasting tin ready and put the kettle on.

2 Pour the milk into a pan with the sugar and vanilla. Bring gently to the boil, stirring to dissolve the sugar. Remove from the heat and cool for a few minutes.

3 In a large bowl, beat the eggs until frothy. Slowly whisk in the cooled milk. Set the ramekins in the roasting tin and divide the custard among them. Pour hot water around the ramekins to come halfway up the sides. Bake for 20 minutes until just set, then cool and chill before serving.

. . . .
PER PUDDING 181 kcals, protein 7g, carbs 28g, fat 5g, sat fat 2g, fibre none, sugar 23g, salt 0.23g

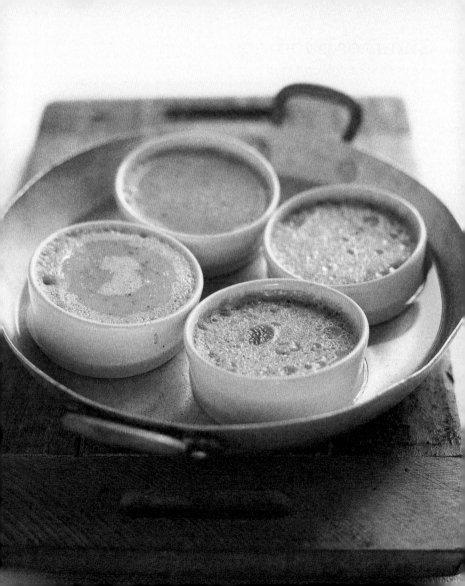

Summer puddings

. . . .

If you have a gluten or wheat intolerance, try these summer puddings made with gluten-free bread. The cut-away bread can be made into breadcrumbs and frozen.

 35 minutes, plus chilling   4

- 250g punnet strawberries, hulled and halved
- 125g punnet blueberries
- 125g punnet blackberries
- 85g/3oz golden caster sugar
- 6 thin slices bread from a gluten-free loaf

1 Put the fruit into a large pan with the sugar and 3 tablespoons water. Heat on low for 2–3 minutes until the juice runs from the fruit. Remove from the heat.

2 Using biscuit cutters, stamp out four 5.5cm circles from the bread, then use a 7-cm cutter for another four circles. Put the smaller circles into the base of four 175ml pudding basins. Spoon in the fruit, then top with the larger circles. Press down, then spoon over just enough juice to colour the bread red, reserving any remaining juice. Cover with cling film and put a weight (such as a jar of jam) on top. Chill for at least 4 hours.

3 To serve the puddings, uncover and run a knife around the edge. Put a serving plate over each one, then invert and spoon over the reserved juice.

. . . .
PER PUDDING 212 kcals, protein 1g, carbs 52g, fat 1g, sat fat none, fibre 2g, sugar 22g, salt 0.53g

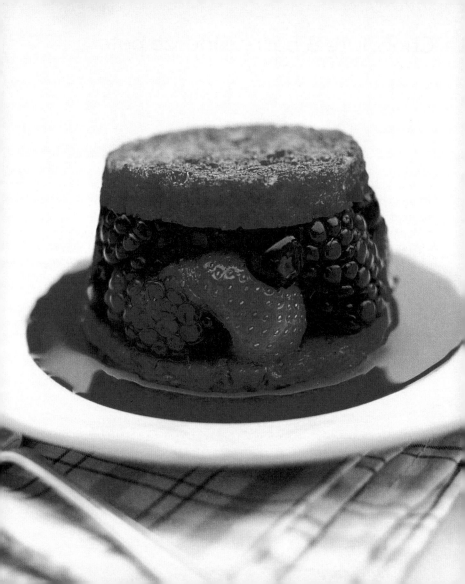

Chocolate & berry mousse pots

. . . .

Dessert doesn't have to be devilish, as this good-for-you pud proves.

🕐 20 minutes   🥧 4

- 75g/2½oz dark chocolate, 70% cocoa solids, grated
- 4 tbsp low-fat natural yogurt
- 2 egg whites
- 2 tsp caster sugar
- 350g/12oz berries (try blueberries, raspberries, cherries or a mix)

1 Melt the chocolate in a heatproof bowl over a pan of simmering water, making sure the bowl doesn't directly touch the water. Once melted, allow it to cool for 5–10 minutes, then stir in the yogurt.

2 Whisk the egg whites in a second bowl until stiff, then whisk in the sugar and beat until stiff again. Fold the whites into the chocolate mix – loosen the mixture first with a spoonful of egg white, then carefully fold in the rest, keeping as much air as possible.

3 Put the berries into four small glasses or ramekins, then spoon the mousse on top. Chill in the fridge until set.

. . . .
PER POT 159 kcals, protein 5g, carbs 19g, fat 8g, sat fat 4g, fibre 3g, sugar 15g, salt 0.13g

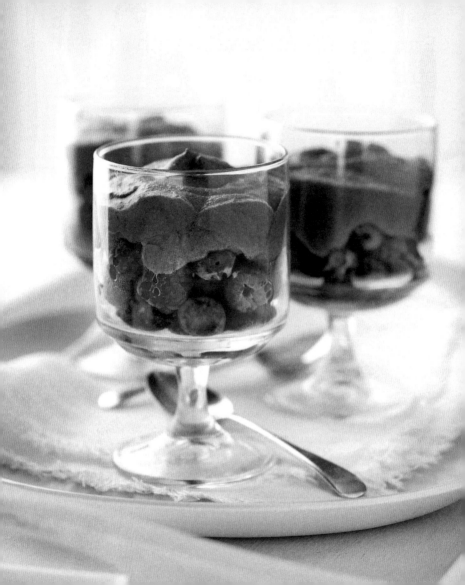

Fromage-frais mousse with strawberry sauce

. . . .

Making this mousse with Italian meringue not only gives you a wonderfully light and airy texture but also means you can serve it to vegetarians, as there is no gelatine.

 25 minutes, plus chilling 6

- 1 egg white
- 50g/2oz icing sugar, plus extra 2 tbsp
- zest 1 lemon and juice ½
- 500g tub low-fat fromage frais
- 500g/1lb 2oz strawberries

1 Put the egg white into a heatproof bowl with the icing sugar. Set the bowl over a large pan of simmering water and, using a hand or electric whisk, whisk for 5 minutes until the mixture is light, fluffy and holds peaks when the blades are lifted. Remove from the heat, whisk in the lemon zest, then whisk for a further 2 minutes to cool it down.

2 Fold in the fromage frais, then transfer the mousse to six glasses or small bowls and chill. Roughly chop half the strawberries and put them in the food processor with the extra 2 tablespoons of the icing sugar and the lemon juice. Whizz to a purée, then press through a sieve to remove the seeds. Chop the remaining strawberries.

3 Spoon the chopped strawberries over the mousses, then spoon a little purée over each. Chill until ready to serve.

. . . .

PER SERVING 118 kcals, protein 8g, carbs 23g, fat none, sat fat none, fibre 1g, sugar 23g, salt 0.13g

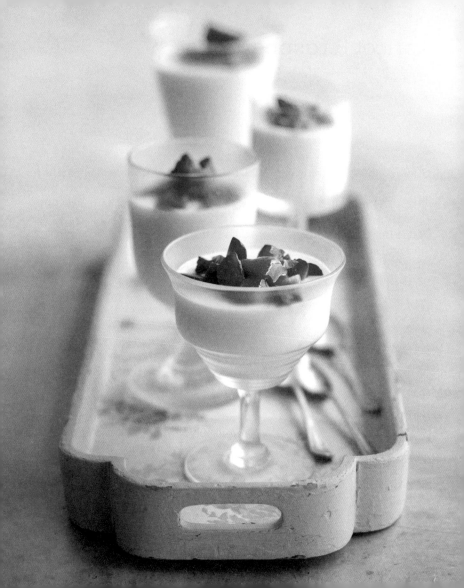

Apricot & raspberry tart

Filo pastry is a low-fat alternative to richer pastries such as shortcrust or puff. However, it needs to be brushed with a little butter as it is layered up.

🕐 40 minutes   🥧 4

- 3 large sheets filo pastry (or 6 small)
- 2 tbsp butter, melted
- 3 tbsp apricot conserve
- 6 ripe apricots, stoned and roughly sliced
- 85g/3oz raspberries
- 2 tsp caster sugar

1 Let the filo come to room temperature for about 10 minutes before use. Put a baking sheet into the oven and heat oven to 200C/180C fan/gas 6.

2 Brush each large sheet of filo with a little of the melted butter, layer on top of each other, then fold in half so you have a smaller rectangle six layers thick. If using small sheets, just brush each with some of the butter and stack them on top of each other. Fold in the edges of the pastry base to make a 2cm/¾in border, then spread the apricot conserve over the pastry sheet inside the border. Carefully slide the pastry base on to the hot baking sheet and bake for 5 minutes.

3 Remove from the oven, arrange the apricots over the tart and brush with any leftover melted butter. Bake for another 10 minutes, then scatter on the raspberries and sprinkle with sugar. Bake for a final 10 minutes until the pastry is golden brown and crisp. Serve warm.

PER SERVING 150 kcals, protein 2g, carbs 22g, fat 7g, sat fat 4g, fibre 2g, sugar 18g, salt 0.33g

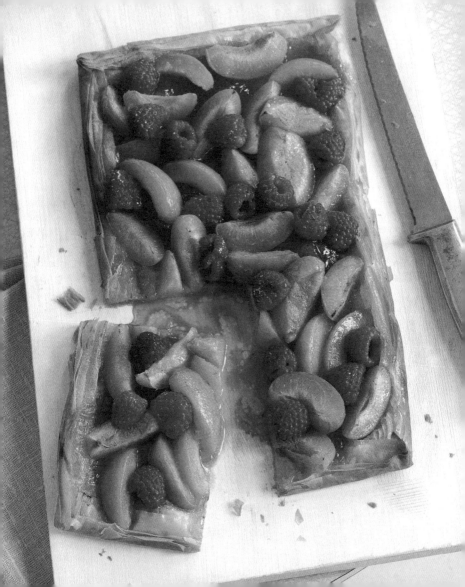

Cherry & raspberry gratin

Make the most of the summer fruits when they're in season. The contrast of sweet vanilla with the tart cherries and raspberries works very well in this healthy pud.

🕐 25 minutes, plus infusing   🍴 4

- 200ml/7fl oz milk
- 1 vanilla pod, split lengthways
- 2 eggs, separated
- 4 tbsp caster sugar
- 1 tbsp plain flour
- squeeze lemon juice
- 300g/10oz stoned cherries
- 300g/10oz raspberries

1 Heat the milk and vanilla pod in a pan until nearly boiling, then leave to infuse for 10–15 minutes. Whisk together the egg yolks with 2 tablespoons of the sugar in a bowl until pale and light, then whisk in the flour to make a paste. Whisk in the warm milk. Pour the custard mixture into clean pan, then cook for 3–5 minutes until thick. Pour through a sieve into a large bowl, discarding the vanilla pod. Leave to cool.

2 Whisk the egg whites until stiff peaks form then add the remaining sugar, a little at a time, whisking well between each addition, until the meringue mixture is thick and glossy. Stir the lemon juice into the custard mix. Add one-third of the meringue to the custard and stir. Repeat with the remaining meringue.

3 Scatter the fruit into a large, shallow heatproof dish. Put under a medium grill for 3–5 minutes to soften. Spoon over the custard-and-meringue mix then grill for 3 minutes until the topping is golden.

PER SERVING 218 kcals, protein 9g, carbs 33g, fat 6g, sat fat 2g, fibre 3g, sugar 30g, salt 0.22g

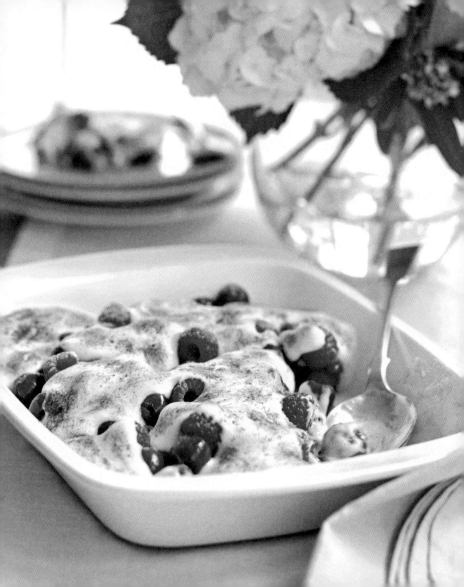

Maple pears with pecans & cranberries

Serve warm for pudding or cool the pears in the fridge overnight, then enjoy with muesli or crunchy oat cereal and yogurt for breakfast.

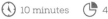 10 minutes 4

- 4 ripe pears
- handful dried cranberries
- 2 tbsp maple syrup, plus extra to drizzle (optional)
- 50g/2oz pecan nuts, roughly chopped
- low-fat Greek yogurt, to serve

1 Peel and halve the pears, and scoop out the core with a teaspoon. Lay the halves in a shallow microwavable dish, cut-side down, along with the cranberries. Pour over the maple syrup over and cover with cling film. Microwave on High for 3 minutes until softened, stirring halfway through. Uncover and leave to cool for a few minutes. Stir the pecan nuts through the syrup.

2 Spoon the fruit and nuts into four serving dishes, drizzle with some extra maple syrup, if you like, and serve with a dollop each of Greek yogurt.

PER SERVING 208 kcals, protein 2g, carbs 32g, fat 9g, sat fat 1g, fibre 4g, sugar 9g, salt none

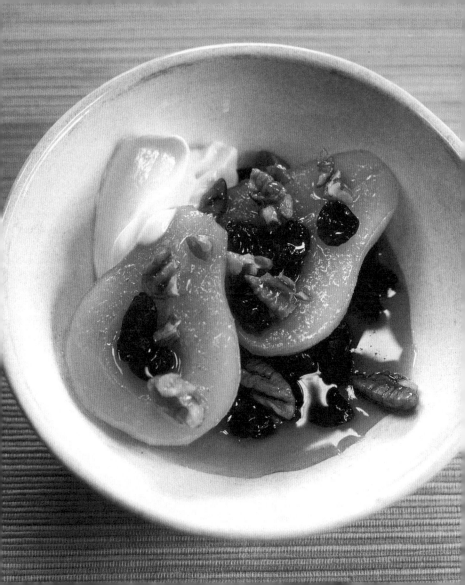

Apple-pie samosas

This sweet version of a savoury favourite makes a tempting hand-held pud. Try other fruits when in season and serve with low-fat yogurt for dipping.

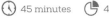 45 minutes   4

- 2 cooking apples, peeled, cored and chopped
- 50g/2oz caster sugar
- 1 tsp ground mixed spice
- 50g/2oz sultanas
- 4 sheets filo pastry
- 25g/1oz low-fat spread, melted
- low-fat natural bio yogurt, to serve (optional)

1 Heat oven to 200C/180C fan/gas 6. Put the apples, sugar, mixed spice and sultanas in a pan with 2 tablespoons water, and cook, covered, for 6 minutes or until the apples are soft, stirring once or twice. Tip into a shallow dish and spread out to cool slightly.

2 Cut the sheets of filo in thirds lengthways, then brush lightly with the melted spread. Put a spoonful of the apple filling at the top of each strip, then fold over and over to form triangular parcels. Put on a baking sheet and bake for 15–20 minutes until crisp and golden. Serve with a dollop of low-fat yogurt, if you like.

PER SERVING 196 kcals, protein 2g, carbs 42g, fat 3g, sat fat 1g, fibre 2g, sugar 31g, salt 0.58g

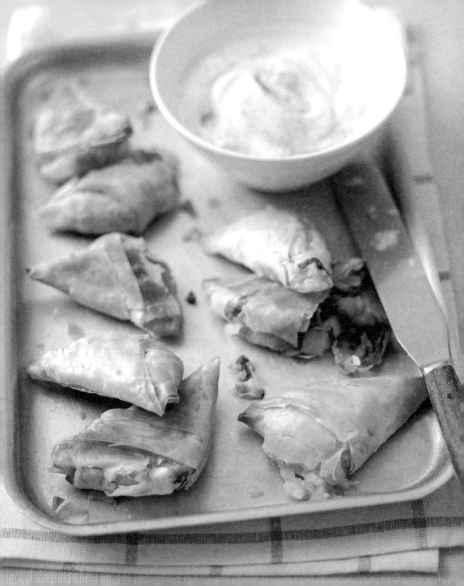

Index

Also available from BBC Books and Good Food

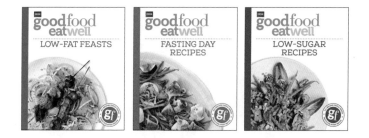

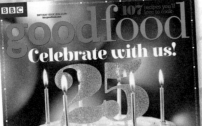